MCQs for MRCOG Part 2

M. A. Khaled MB BS LMSSA MRCOG
Senior Registrar
Hope Hospital
Salford

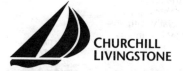

CHURCHILL
LIVINGSTONE

EDINBURGH LONDON MADRID MELBOURNE NEW YORK
SAN FRANCISCO AND TOKYO 1998

CHURCHILL LIVINGSTONE
Medical Division of Pearson Professional Limited

Distributed in the United States of America by Churchill
Livingstone Inc., 650 Avenue of the Americas, New York,
N.Y. 10011, and by associated companies, branches and
representatives throughout the world.

First published 1998

ISBN 0443 06122X

British Library of Cataloguing in Publication Data
A catalogue record for this book is available from the
British Library.

Library of Congress Cataloging in Publication Data
A catalog record for this book is available from the
Library of Congress.

Medical knowledge is constantly changing. As information
becomes available, changes in treatment, procedures,
equipment and the use of drugs become necessary. The
author and publisher have, as far as it is possible, taken
care to ensure that the information given in the text is
accurate and up-to-date. However, readers are strongly
advised to confirm that the information, especially with
regard to drug usage, complies with current legislation
and standard of practice.

The
publisher's
policy is to use
paper manufactured
from sustainable forests

Produced by Longman Asia Ltd, Hong Kong
EPC/01

Contents

Preface   vii

The MRCOG exam   ix

Questions   1

Answers   67

Preface

Adequate exam preparation is always a difficult task for candidates and the MCQ component provides an additional challenge. The Royal College of Obstetricians and Gynaecologists has maintained the lead in modifying exam format and the new form of MCQ, as shown in this text, matches that set by the College. The style of numbering the questions in this book has been altered slightly to make the answers easier to identify.

In this undertaking, there are a number of individuals who deserve recognition and my gratitude. First, I would like to thank Dr Angela Railton, for her excellent, timely and well-researched contribution to this book, and Mr Roger Jackson, the Examinations Secretary of the Royal College of Obstetricians and Gynaecologists, who advised on the text and gave the College's permission to include the standard format given to all candidates. I would also like to thank Miss Christine Laing for typing the text and for her tireless efforts and senses of responsibility and humour, which kept me going in moments of despair. Finally, I would like to thank my family for their continuous support.

Whilst every effort has been made to check each question in the text, from current textbooks and recent journals, some answers may be slightly controversial. The view expressed is my own and I take responsibility for it. The idea is to encourage readers to review the literature to get the correct answer as seen by the candidate. This is, of course, the main objective of such a text: to encourage the candidate to research many topics prior to the written exam. There are gaps in the knowledge of anyone who prepares for any exam and this book is intended to help all candidates fill these gaps.

I hope the average candidate will find it as expected and I would value comments on it.

1998   M. A. Khaled

The MRCOG exam

The following is an extract from the MCQ instructions from the
Royal College of Obstetricians and Gynaecologists.

Answering the questions
The Answer Sheet is numbered 1–300 and against each number
there are two lozenges labelled T (= True) and F (= False). You
will be required to indicate whether you know a particular
question to.be true or false by boldly blacking out either the
True or False lozenge.

To avoid too many erasures on the Answer Sheet, candidates
may wish to mark their responses in the Question Book and
then transfer their decisions to the Answer Sheet but this must
be done within the two hours allowed for the examination.

Specimen questions and answers

When compared with radiotherapy, radical hysterectomy:

1. is less favoured in stage 1a carcinoma of the cervix
2. carries a reduced risk of subsequent lymphocyst
    formation
3. allows preservation of ovarian function

Uterine curettage:

4. is associated with an increased incidence of placenta
    praevia in a subsequent pregnancy
5. is important in the investigation of secondary infertility

Ovarian thecomata:

6. are typically benign

The following genital anomalies have a recognized association with the conditions listed:

7. hypospadias: androgen insensitivity (testicular feminization syndrome)
8. hypertrophy of the clitoris: maternal nortestosterone therapy
9. varicocele: Klinefelter's syndrome

In a patient with inappropriate lactation associated with secondary amenorrhoea:

10. bitemporal hemianopia on perimetry would be expected in about 25% of patients
11. an exaggerated rise in serum prolactin concentration following infection of thyrotrophin-releasing hormone is a recognized finding
12. an increased plasma concentration would be expected
13. treatment with Danazol would be appropriate
14. the administration of methyldopa is a recognized cause
15. anorexia nervosa is a recognized association

Answers 3, 6, 8, 11 and 14 are 'True'; answers 1, 2, 4, 5, 7, 9, 10, 12, 13 and 15 are 'False'.

Marking
Each question correctly answered (i.e. a true statement indicated as True or a false statement indicated as False) is awarded one mark (+1). For each incorrect answer no mark (0) is awarded. All questions must be answered true or false. Incorrect answers are not penalized.

QUESTIONS

1. **The following relate to placenta praevia:**

   A. it is commoner in primigravidae
   B. it carries an increased risk of intrauterine growth retardation (IUGR)
   C. the incidence of postpartum haemorrhage is increased
   D. it is commoner in women who have undergone a myomectomy
   E. posterior placenta praevia is easier to diagnose sonographically

2. **Known biochemical screening methods for Down's syndrome include:**

   A. alpha feto protein
   B. human chorionic gonadotrophin
   C. serum progesterone
   D. unconjugated oestriol
   E. urea-resistant neutrophil alkaline phosphatase
   F. inhibin A
   G. follicular-stimulating hormone
   H. pregnancy-associated placental protein
   I. urinary gonadotrophin peptide

3. **The following are not contraindications to the use of combined oral contraception (COC):**

   A. pemphigoid gestationalis
   B. ischaemic heart disease
   C. liver adenoma
   D. focal migraine
   E. chorea

4. **Placenta accreta:**

   A. is a placenta attached, either partly or completely, directly to the uterine muscle
   B. is unlikely in a patient who has suffered from Ashermann's syndrome
   C. has a predisposing factor of chronic endometritis
   D. is managed most safely by hysterectomy
   E. is commonly associated with placenta praevia

5. **Thecomas:**

   A. occur in all age groups
   B. are usually cystic
   C. are usually bilateral
   D. are essentially benign lesions

6. **The following are contraindications to the use of progesterone-only pills (POPs):**

   A. peptic ulcer
   B. previous PID
   C. a history of ovarian cysts
   D. active liver disease
   E. bottle feeding
   F. endometriosis

7. **Behavioural therapies in cases of detrusor instability include:**

   A. hypnotherapy
   B. bladder drill
   C. acupuncture
   D. biofeedback
   E. Burch colposuspension

8. **Cis platin:**

   A. has an alkylating action
   B. is given intramuscularly
   C. has no effect on the kidneys
   D. can cause autotoxicity
   E. can cause peripheral neuropathy
   F. can cause hypermagnesaemia

9. **With regard to cytomegalovirus infection:**
   A. cytomegaloviruses are related to the herpes group of viruses
   B. cytomegalovirus infection in pregnancy is characterized by a large-for-dates uterus
   C. cytomegalovirus transmission is restricted to the first and second trimester
   D. recurrent maternal infection may affect the fetus
   E. routine antenatal screening includes screening for cytomegalovirus

10. **The following relate to ovarian tumours in pregnancy:**
    A. laparotomy in the first trimester is indicated in the majority of cases
    B. benign cystic teratoma is the commonest tumour
    C. about 10% of ovarian tumours occurring in pregnancy are malignant

11. **With regard to vaginosis:**
    A. bacterial vaginosis is a clinical syndrome in which *Lactobacillus* is replaced by *Gardnerella vaginalis* and/or *Mycoplasma hominis*
    B. bacterial vaginosis has a link with cellulitis of the vaginal cuff following hysterectomy
    C. bacterial vaginosis is not associated with pelvic inflammatory disease
    D. clindamycin is the treatment of choice in cases of bacterial vaginosis and may be given safely during pregnancy
    E. women with bacterial vaginosis are twice as likely to have infection of the placental membrane

12. **The following statements are correct:**
    A. leiomyomata are the commonest tumours of the round ligament
    B. intraligamentous fibromyoma is not an uncommon broad ligament tumour
    C. Gartner's duct may be the origin of a broad ligament cyst

13. **The following relate to fallopian tube tumours:**
  A. previous ectopic pregnancy is a recognized risk factor
  B. papillary adenocarcinoma is the commonest primary tumour
  C. they are unlikely to be of metastatic origin
  D. the 5-year survival rate for tubal cancer is 60–80%
  E. they rarely present with profuse vaginal discharge

14. **In early development:**
  A. the amnion is a double layer of fetal mesodermal origin
  B. the decidua capsularis is a component of the chorion
  C. chorionic villi are the functional hormonal units
  D. human chorionic gonadotrophin is produced mainly by cytotrophoblasts
  E. relaxin is produced by the corpus luteum and the decidua

15. **The following methods are used for investigating the fallopian tubes:**
  A. mucosal biopsy
  B. salpingoscopy
  C. bacteriological investigation
  D. tubal fluid sampling
  E. sperm transport
  F. dilatation and cutterage (D&C)

16. **The following drugs are known to interact with COCs:**
  A. barbiturates
  B. rifampicin
  C. non-steroidal anti-inflammatories
  D. chloroquine
  E. insulin
  F. aspirin

17. **Papillomaviruses:**
    A. are considered as one genus of the Papovaviridae family
    B. are single-stranded RNA viruses

18. **With regard to umbilical vessels:**
    A. normally there are two arteries and one vein
    B. a single umbilical artery is found in 5% of all singleton pregnancies
    C. a single umbilical artery is common in diabetic mothers
    D. a single umbilical artery is commonly associated with an absent corpus callosum

19. **With regard to transverse vaginal septa:**
    A. the minority of these occur at the junction of the middle and upper two-thirds of the vagina
    B. concurrent endometriosis may hamper the success of surgery
    C. Williams' vulvovaginoplasty is indicated

20. **A large placenta has an association with:**
    A. hypertensive disorders of pregnancy
    B. maternal anaemia
    C. ABO incompatibility
    D. fetal lung malformation
    E. alpha thalassaemia
    F. syphilis

21. **In chorion villus sampling:**
    A. rapid cytogenic results may be obtained within 4 hours
    B. fetal loss occurs in 7%
    C. severe limb deformities occur if performed before 66 days' gestation
    D. chorionic sample always matches fetal karyotype

22. **The following should be considered in postmature pregnancy:**
    A. wrong dates
    B. fetal adrenal hyperplasia
    C. placental sulfatase deficiency
    D. extrauterine pregnancy
    E. maternal hypothyroidism

23. **The following relate to herpes genitalis:**
    A. initial herpes genitalis infection is always symptomatic
    B. about one-third of the population may show serological evidence of herpes without symptoms
    C. Acyclovir is the only absorbable agent used for treating herpes
    D. serum creatinine should be checked in patients receiving high dosage Acyclovir
    E. HPV types 6 and 11 are known to carry oncogenic risks
    F. the vast majority of HPV infections are related to sexual behaviour
    G. children may contract non-genital-type HPV-containing verrucae (Type 2) in their perianal or vulval skin from their parents
    H. herpes is a single-stranded DNA virus
    I. Lichen nitidus is another name for HPV
    J. the incidence of HPV infection has a direct correlation with the number of sexual partners

24. **With regard to HIV infections:**

    A. HIV infections are often multicentric
    B. in women who are HIV positive, the incidence of pelvic inflammatory disease is increased
    C. there is an increased risk of CIN in a patient who is HIV positive
    D. oligomenorrhoea and amenorrhoea are predominant symptoms in HIV-positive patients
    E. oestradiol levels fall with advanced HIV disease
    F. pregnancy accelerates the clinical course of HIV
    G. latex condoms are effective in preventing the transmission of HIV
    H. combined oral contraceptive pills are contraindicated in an HIV-positive woman
    I. the intrauterine contraceptive device (IUCD) is the ideal contraceptive for a woman with HIV
    J. a woman who is HIV positive has a 10% chance of developing AIDS in 5 years

25. **With regard to COC:**

    A. premenstrual syndrome may be aggravated
    B. there is a 50% reduction in the incidence of pelvic inflammatory disease
    C. there is an increase in the incidence of ectopic pregnancy
    D. there is a 50% reduction in the incidence of benign functional ovarian cysts
    E. there is a 50% reduction in the risk of developing endometrial cancer

26. **The following are characteristic of a normal semen analysis:**

    A. more than 50% of spermatozoa have normal morphology
    B. there are more than 1×10^6/ml white blood cells
    C. there is at least 10 mg of citric acid per ejaculate
    D. there is at least 2.4 µmol of calcium per ejaculate

27. **With regard to vaginitis:**

    A. profuse, malodorous and greenish discharge are characteristic features of trichomonal vaginitis

    B. *Trichomonas vaginalis* is multicellular and flagellated

    C. clue cells may point to the diagnosis of trichomonal vaginitis

    D. metronidazole is the drug of choice for trichomonal vaginitis

    E. *Trichomonas vaginalis* may be a cause of pelvic inflammatory disease

    F. atrophic vaginitis occurs only in postmenopausal women

    G. secondary bacterial infection is common in women with atrophic vaginitis

    H. atrophic vaginitis may interfere with the interpretation of cervical cytology

    I. itching is a common symptom in women with atrophic vaginitis

    J. vaginal bleeding does not occur in patients with atrophic vaginitis

28. **In a pregnant woman who has HIV:**

    A. there is an increased risk of perinatal death

    B. immune function tests should be performed every 3 months

    C. weight loss is a significant factor in predicting pregnancy outcome

    D. *Toxoplasma gondii* is an unlikely association

29. **The following relate to pelvic inflammatory disease (PID):**

    A. it is common in early pregnancy

    B. the incidence of PID is higher in women who use barrier methods of contraception

    C. oral contraceptives render the patient more susceptible to PID

    D. chlamydial infection is a recognized risk factor in PID

    E. infection may follow intrauterine insemination

    F. midcycle is the most common time for infection

    G. a history of laparoscopic sterilization precludes the diagnosis of PID

30. **The following are associated with fetal macrosomia:**

    A. maternal obesity
    B. maternal diabetes insipidus
    C. maternal toxoplasmosis
    D. previous macrosomic baby

31. **The following are characteristic features of Edward's syndrome:**

    A. single umbilical artery
    B. long sternum
    C. rocker bottom feet
    D. hydrocephalus
    E. trisomy 13

32. **Spermatogenesis is affected by:**

    A. cimetidine
    B. tetracycline
    C. nitrofurantoin
    D. hypothermia
    E. metronidazole

33. **With regard to amniotic fluid:**

    A. the maximum volume can be seen at 32–36 weeks' gestation
    B. the volume at term is about 200 ml
    C. oligohydramnios tends to be related to IUGR and postmaturity
    D. infantile polycystic kidneys are associated with polyhydramnios
    E. cord compression is associated with polyhydramnios

34. **Elevated serum alpha feto protein is associated with:**

    A. maternal diabetes mellitus
    B. multiple pregnancy
    C. maternal obesity
    D. omphalocele

35. **The following are associated with multiple pregnancy:**

    A. discordant growth
    B. decreased incidence of abruption and placenta praevia
    C. cephalic/cephalic presentation occurs in about 70%
    D. induction of labour is advisable as a routine procedure at 38 weeks

36. **The following are classified as epithelial cell tumours of the ovary:**

    A. gonadoblastoma
    B. endometrioid tumours
    C. clear cell tumours
    D. granulosa cell tumour
    E. dysgerminoma

37. **The following relate to intrauterine growth retardation:**

    A. asymmetrical IUGR is seen with intrauterine infection
    B. malnutrition may lead to asymmetrical IUGR
    C. severe anaemia is associated with symmetrical IUGR

38. **The following relate to emergency contraceptive methods:**

    A. RU486 produces its action through changes in the tubal epithelium
    B. for the IUCD to be effective, it should be inserted within 5 days of intercourse
    C. as emergency contraception, the IUCD has a failure rate of 6%
    D. progestogen alone is not a suitable emergency contraception

39. **The following are complications of cocaine during pregnancy:**

    A. placenta praevia
    B. increased spontaneous abortion in up to 40% of cases
    C. significant postmaturity
    D. increased incidence of skeletal defects
    E. sudden infant death syndrome in about 10–15%

40. **Cardiac diseases that are known to lead to an increased maternal mortality include:**
    A. Marfan's syndrome
    B. cardiomyopathy
    C. pulmonary hypertension
    D. ventricular septal defect

41. **The following relate to hyperemesis gravidarum:**
    A. it may lead to preterm labour
    B. there is a recognized risk of maternal death
    C. it is associated with Wernicke's encephalitis
    D. it is commoner in IVF pregnancies

42. **The following are common neonatal complications in babies born to diabetic mums:**
    A. respiratory distress syndrome
    B. hyperglycaemia
    C. hypercalcaemia
    D. polycythemia
    E. hypobilirubinaemia

43. **Contraceptive implants:**
    A. contain levonorgestrel
    B. are effective for 15 years
    C. may be inserted on the seventh day following termination of pregnancy
    D. are not suitable for obese women
    E. cause menstrual abnormalities in about 20% of users

44. **In gestational diabetes:**
    A. 25–40% of gestational diabetic women will develop diabetes mellitus later in life
    B. all patients with gestational diabetes should have insulin
    C. a history of recurrent candida may be the early symptom
    D. pregnancies should be induced at 38 weeks

45. **The following relate to ovulation:**

A. it occurs approximately 18 hours after the LH peak
B. it occurs 24–36 hours after the peak oestradiol level has been obtained
C. the LH peak occurs 34–36 hours after follicular rupture
D. a rise in intrafollicular concentration of plasmin stimulates proteolytic enzymes
E. inhibition of prostaglandin synthesis within the follicle leads to luteinized unruptured follicle syndrome

46. **The following are true for rubella:**

A. it has a regular periodicity similar to measles
B. it has an incubation period of 7–14 days

47. **The following relate to the intrauterine contraceptive device:**

A. it has a protective effect against ectopic pregnancy directly proportional to the surface area of copper in the IUCD
B. it is expelled less in younger patients
C. it is associated with a uterine perforation rate of 2.4–4 per 1000 during insertion
D. peritoneal placement may be treated conservatively with repeat ultrasound
E. the risk of infection is highest in the first weeks after insertion

48. **The following are associated with low blood pressure in early pregnancy:**

A. hydatidiform mole
B. renal disease
C. cocaine abuse
D. triploidy

49. **The following relate to hydatidiform mole:**

    A. the complete mole arises from fertilization of an empty ovum
    B. in the complete mole, half the chromosomes are paternally derived
    C. the commonest chromosome in the complete mole is 45XY
    D. the usual chromosome pattern in the partial mole is a triploidy
    E. partial hydatidiform chromosomes are paternally derived
    F. there is a 15–20% malignant potential in the partial mole
    G. 2–3% of complete moles will progress to choriocarcinoma

50. **In barrier methods of contraception:**

    A. the male condom, if used carefully, has a failure rate of one pregnancy per 100 couple years
    B. lubrication with an oil-based substance does not interfere with the efficacy of the male condom
    C. the latex rubber of the condom transfers body heat
    D. the female condom is frequently lubricated with spermicide

51. **Sensory urgency may be caused by:**

    A. UTI
    B. interstitial cystitis
    C. squamous cell carcinoma of the bladder
    D. bladder stones
    E. an idiopathic cause

52. **The following are characteristic features of Sheehan's syndrome:**

    A. postural hypotension
    B. occurrence of symptoms immediately after delivery
    C. excessive milk production
    D. symptoms of hyperthyroidism

53. **In placental site trophoblastic tumour:**

   A. serum hCG is usually high
   B. the response to chemotherapy is poor
   C. surgery is the main form of therapy
   D. villi are characteristically increased
   E. a low serum human placental lactogen is characteristic

54. **With regard to Turner's syndrome:**

   A. it is characterized by non-pitting oedema at birth
   B. the incidence is 1 in 2500 live births
   C. it may occur either in the pure or mosaic form
   D. positive sex chromatin is a feature
   E. there is a high oestrogen level
   F. mosaicism can occur only after fertilization
   G. aortic incompetence is a feature

55. **The following relate to Klinefelter's syndrome:**

   A. the defect is in the meiotic division of the sperm and ovum
   B. there is an extra sex chromosome
   C. testicular volume usually exceeds 4 ml
   D. individuals usually have a large prostate
   E. oligospermia is a characteristic feature

56. **With regard to the urethral syndrome:**

   A. there are symptoms of frequency and dysuria in the presence of bacteriuria
   B. there is detrusor instability, with generalized or local disease excluded
   C. symptoms are rarely seen before puberty
   D. symptoms usually follow a cyclical pattern, with periods of remission
   E. symptoms are not related to the menstrual cycle
   F. diurnal frequency is a constant symptom

57.   **The contraceptive diaphragm (cap):**

   A. is available in different sizes from 40 to 120 mm
   B. can be inserted at any time after intercourse
   C. should remain in place for at least 2 hours after intercourse
   D. may lead to urinary symptoms
   E. has higher failure rates than other methods

58.   **Uterine leiomyomata:**

   A. may be associated with polycythemia and hypertension
   B. may be the cause of early pregnancy loss
   C. are treated by myomectomy as the treatment of choice in the majority of cases
   D. are complicated by sarcomatous lesions in 3% of cases
   E. recur in 30% of cases following myomectomy

59.   **The following may cause second trimester miscarriage:**

   A. asthma
   B. mullerian fusion abnormality
   C. *Toxoplasma gondii*
   D. *Listeria monocytogenes*
   E. malaria
   F. aspirin
   G. syphilis
   H. systemic lupus erythematosus
   I. thyrotoxicosis

60.   **The following relate to dysmenorrhoea:**

   A. childbirth has a curative effect on secondary dysmenorrhoea
   B. in the presence of endometriosis, the pain increases throughout menstruation
   C. pain prior to menstruation suggests PID

61. **The following relate to postcoital contraceptive pills:**

    A. they contain 100 µg ethinyloestradiol and 0.5 mg levonorgestrel
    B. Yuzpe is recommended for use within 3 days of unprotected intercourse
    C. they may lead to severe nausea
    D. the failure rate is independent of the stage of the menstrual cycle
    E. they may be used on a woman with a history of migraine

62. **The following are complications of pelvic inflammatory disease:**

    A. recurrent pelvic abscess
    B. infertility
    C. perihepatitis
    D. menorrhagia
    E. depression

63. **The following are used to treat fibroids:**

    A. progesterone antagonists
    B. Danazol
    C. GnRH antagonists
    D. Heparin
    E. HRT therapy

64. **The following are contraindications to the use of the IUCD as a method of contraception:**

    A. a partner who is HIV positive
    B. the presence of valvular heart disease
    C. previous ectopic pregnancy
    D. the presence of a fundal fibroid of more than 2 cm diameter
    E. hypothyroidism

65. **Abnormal uterine bleeding may be due to:**
    A. irritable bowel syndrome
    B. adenomyosis
    C. hyperthyroidism
    D. hypothyroidism
    E. Von Willebrand's disease
    F. adult phenylketonuria
    G. migraine

66. **The following relate to menorrhagia:**
    A. it is usually associated with iron deficiency anaemia
    B. 5% of women below 40 present with this symptom
    C. D&C is the most accurate diagnostic tool

67. **With regard to colposcopy:**
    A. colposcopy was first introduced by Hinselmann in 1960
    B. iodine is used to identify glycogen-containing areas
    C. it is considered an effective screening method for cervical carcinoma
    D. the green filter is used mainly for blood vessels, especially in early invasion
    E. cervicography is used to increase the sensitivity of the technique

68. **The following relate to Bartholin's glands:**
    A. they secrete mucus maximally at the time of menstruation
    B. secretion drains to the posterior introitus
    C. abscesses should be treated initially with antibiotics
    D. abscesses are most commonly caused by streptococcal infection

69. **The following are true for dysmenorrhoea:**
    A. the secondary type will always have an underlying aetiology
    B. physical examination is often helpful
    C. contraceptive pills are of limited value in treatment
    D. transcutaneous electrical nerve stimulation may be of help in treatment

70. **The following relate to *lichen sclerosis et atrophicus***
    A. it involves the pudendum either partially or completely
    B. it may be mistaken for morphoea
    C. it does not affect the skin surrounding the anus
    D. the lesion is usually thick and white with crinkly plaques
    E. it may involve the trunk or limbs in 1% of patients
    F. epidermal hypertrophy is a characteristic feature
    G. epidermal hyalinization is a feature
    H. there is a correlation between the histology and the clinical features
    I. it is of autoimmune aetiology
    J. a reduced serum dihydrotestosterone and androstenedione may indicate poor prognosis
    K. vulval carcinoma may occur in the presence of lichen sclerosis
    L. treatment may involve bland emollient creams
    M. steroids may produce more thinning and atrophy

71. **With regard to dermatosis of the vulva:**
    A. *Lichen simplex chronicus* does not occur in normal skin
    B. *Lichen planus* may lead to adhesions and vaginal stenosis
    C. contact dermatitis may result from partner's sperm
    D. steroids are not effective in cases of vulval psoriasis
    E. sedation at night may be helpful in some cases of vulval diseases

72. **The following relate to neural tube defects (NTDs):**
    A. there are genetic and environmental factors associated with the aetiology
    B. there is a relation to poor nutrition
    C. recurrence is around 10%
    D. they are likely to occur more in women who suffer from severe megaloblastic anaemia

73. **The following are characteristic features of antiphospholipid antibody syndrome:**

    A. recurrent miscarriages
    B. severe fetal growth retardation
    C. large placental infarcts
    D. venous thrombosis
    E. a lower risk of pregnancy loss with a new partner

74. **Uterine fibroids:**

    A. are composed of striated muscle and connective tissue
    B. are more common in Caucasians than Africans
    C. are unaffected by GnRH analogue
    D. may cause ureteric obstruction

75. **The following relate to postnatal depression:**

    A. about 10–15% of women are depressed within 12 months of childbirth
    B. age and parity are associated with an increased risk
    C. operative delivery is not associated with an increased risk
    D. initial insomnia may be the first indication of the depression
    E. anhedonia is accompanied by loss of libido

76. **Imperforate hymen:**

    A. may lead to haematosalpinx
    B. is usually identified earlier in life than at puberty
    C. is frequently associated with renal abnormalities
    D. is often found with uterus didelphis
    E. generally requires reconstructive surgery

77. **With regard to diverticulae of the urethra:**

A. burning micturition suggests infection
B. dribbling of urine and a sensation of incomplete bladder emptying are common symptoms
C. the diagnosis is made clinically in the majority of cases
D. surgical treatment is indicated in the presence of diverticulae
E. this is the origin of urethral caruncles

78. **Urethral caruncles:**

A. are granulomatous lesions
B. are precursors of urethral cancer
C. usually protrude from the edges of the urethra
D. may be mistaken for prolapsed urethral mucosa
E. once diagnosed, should always be treated

79. **The following relate to pelvic floor laxity:**

A. an enterocoele is a prolapse of the rectum into the vagina
B. levator ani are the most important ligaments supporting the pelvis
C. vaginal atrophy is a common cause in cases of cystocoele
D. it is associated with a high body mass index
E. rectocoeles require treatment in all cases to prevent enterocoele formation

80. **With regard to genuine stress incontinence (GSI):**

A. it occurs when the maximum urethral pressure exceeds the intravesical pressure
B. it is commoner in women between the ages of 25 and 65
C. surgery remains the most effective therapy
D. Burch colposuspension may be performed when there is a foreshortened, scarred and immobile vagina

81. **Irreversible causes of delayed puberty in girls include:**

    A. anorexia nervosa
    B. hyperprolactinaemia
    C. hypothyroidism
    D. Kallman's syndrome
    E. diabetes mellitus

82. **The following relate to incontinence:**

    A. it is frequently associated with cystourethrocoele in females
    B. urge incontinence is more frequent than GSI
    C. the angle between the bladder and the urethra is narrowed in cases of GSI
    D. female urinary incontinence is always related to underlying pathology

83. **GnRH analogue therapy is of value in the treatment of:**

    A. uterine fibroids
    B. adenomyosis
    C. premenstrual tension syndrome
    D. hypoandrogenic state
    E. dysfunctional uterine bleeding

84. **With regard to 6 months of therapy with GnRH analogue:**

    A. it is associated with an 8% reduction of bone density in the spine
    B. it is associated with a 10% reduction of bone density in the hip
    C. the reduction in bone density is reversible once the drug is discontinued
    D. add-back therapy may avoid reduction in bone density
    E. the treatment may be extended for a further 6 months

85. **A natural menopause:**

A. occurs earlier in smokers
B. occurs later than average in nulliparous compared to parous women
C. can only be defined retrospectively
D. commonly has mood change as the first symptom
E. occurs significantly earlier in black women

86. **The following relate to the menopause:**

A. it is characterized by a daily loss of calcium
B. it is associated with high levels of plasma calcitonin
C. it is associated with a fall in alkaline phosphate levels
D. it commonly occurs earlier in women with liver disease
E. HRT is the commonest cause of postmenopausal bleeding

87. **Premature ovarian failure:**

A. occurs in 15% of women
B. is unlikely to occur prior to puberty
C. may be caused by previous surgery
D. is unlikely to be caused by infection
E. should be confirmed by ovarian biopsy

88. **With regard to postoperative catheterization:**

A. it carries a risk of infection of about 40–60% with a Foley catheter
B. a suprapubic catheter is associated with a 15–20% risk of infection
C. it is not required for Burch colposuspension

89. **Hysteroscopy:**

A. has a role in the investigation of infertility
B. may be used to perform sterilization
C. can be performed if the patient suffers mild pelvic inflammatory disease
D. may be complicated by endometritis
E. is always performed under general anaesthetic

90. With regard to COCs:

- **A.** mild diarrhoea affects the efficacy of the pill
- **B.** the failure rate is about 0.2–0.3 per 100 women years
- **C.** about 40% of women will experience a reduction in their monthly menstrual flow
- **D.** the primary mode of action is by inhibition of ovulation

91. The following relate to prematurity:

- **A.** cervical incompetence is beneficial only in 1 out of 25 cases at high risk for preterm labour
- **B.** a maternal age of below 20 is not a risk factor
- **C.** preterm labour is commoner in multiparous women
- **D.** decidual vasculopathy is a recognized cause of preterm delivery
- **E.** prematurity remains the commonest cause of neonatal death in the normally formed baby

92. Progesterone only contraceptive pills:

- **A.** include ethynodiol diacetate
- **B.** have no effect on the function of the fallopian tubes
- **C.** have failure rates of 3 to 7 pregnancies per 100 women years
- **D.** have an adverse effect on lactation
- **E.** are contraindicated in diabetes mellitus

93. Depot medroxyprogesterone acetate:

- **A.** is a derivative of 19-alpha-hydroxyprogesterone
- **B.** has no action on the fallopian tubes
- **C.** is affected by liver enzyme-inducing agents
- **D.** improves premenstrual tension syndrome

94. **The following are true for normal vaginal discharge:**

    A. it consists of uterine and vaginal secretions
    B. normal vaginal pH is 3.8–4.2
    C. itching may be considered a normal phenomenon in physiological vaginal discharge
    D. the amount of physiological vaginal discharge varies with the day of the menstrual cycle
    E. Doderlein's bacillus is an anaerobic gram-positive rod

95. **The following medical conditions are not aggravated by the use of the combined oral contraceptive pill:**

    A. asthma
    B. multiple sclerosis
    C. systemic lupus erythematosus
    D. rheumatoid arthritis
    E. sarcoidosis

96. **The following relate to female sterilization:**

    A. the partner's consent is essential
    B. it is associated with a failure rate of 1–2%
    C. hysterectomy may be the method of choice in some cases
    D. sterilization during Caesarean section carries the same failure rate as an elective procedure

97. **The following medications are known for their teratogenic effects:**

    A. danazol
    B. warfarin
    C. aspirin
    D. phenytoin
    E. temazepam

98. **The following relate to deep vein thrombosis (DVT) in pregnancy:**

    A. the incidence of DVT in all pregnancies is 0.5–1.4%
    B. DVT in pregnancy is three times greater in the right leg than in the left
    C. sickle cell trait has an association with venous thrombosis in pregnancy
    D. ultrasound scanning may be accurate in diagnosing DVT in the calf
    E. antiphospholipid antibody syndrome is associated with chorea gravidarum and DVT
    F. the average life span for platelets is between 30 and 45 days
    G. warfarin may cause alopecia, thrombocytopenia and osteoporosis

99. **The following drugs may be associated with unwanted side-effects in a breast-fed baby:**

    A. carbimazole
    B. erythromycin
    C. indomethacin
    D. benzodiazepines
    E. methyldopa

100. **With regard to toxoplasmosis in pregnancy:**

    A. it is always symptomatic in the woman
    B. it has an incidence of 2% in the UK
    C. hydrocephalus is an associated complication
    D. transmission is 50% in the first trimester
    E. diagnosis is made by the demonstration of toxoplasma-specific IgG

101. **The following may influence male fertility:**

    A. diabetes insipidus
    B. bronchitis
    C. urinary tract infection
    D. unilateral maldescent of the testes
    E. excessive alcohol consumption

102. **The following relate to CIN and cervical neoplasia:**

    A. all invasive squamous cell carcinomas of the cervix are preceded by CIN

    B. for CIN to progress to an invasive lesion may take up to 10 years

    C. Epstein–Barr, hepatitis B and HTLV-1 are linked strongly to the development of cervical neoplasia

    D. if colposcopy is unsatisfactory and the smear shows severe dyskaryosis, hysterectomy is indicated

    E. CIN III will progress to invasive disease in 0.3–0.4% of cases, despite cone biopsy or hysterectomy

    F. cervical stenosis following cone biopsy is always symptomatic

103. **With regard to vascular disease in pregnancy:**

    A. cerebrovascular disease is five times more common during pregnancy and the puerperium

    B. antithrombin III, protein c and protein s are all vitamin-K-dependent factors

    C. about 30% of women with hereditary antithrombin III develop a venous thrombosis in pregnancy

    D. there is a clinical association between antiphospholipid antibody syndrome and cerebrovascular disease

    E. in compensated DIC, the platelet count, fibrinogen level and PTT may be normal

    F. pulmonary embolism occurs in 12% of all pregnancies

104. **Granulosa cell tumours:**

    A. account for 10% of all solid malignant ovarian neoplasms

    B. do not occur before puberty

    C. may result in precocious puberty

    D. are associated with endometrial hyperplasia

    E. have a poor prognosis

    F. are associated with endometrial adenocarcinoma in 20% of cases

105. **The following relate to ectopic pregnancy:**

    A. there is an increased risk of ectopic pregnancy with IVF and embryo transfer
    B. in ectopic pregnancy, abdominal pain is present in about 60% of cases
    C. current IUCD, infertility and PID are risk factors for ectopic pregnancy
    D. ectopic pregnancy is associated with normal corpus luteum function
    E. a coexisting ectopic and intrauterine pregnancy occurs in 1 in 3000 pregnancies
    F. laparoscopy provides the diagnosis of ectopic pregnancy in about 90% of cases
    G. methotrexate, prostaglandin F2a α and hyperosmolar glucose are known treatments for ectopic pregnancy
    H. diethylstilbestrol (DES) exposure is a risk factor for ectopic pregnancy

106. **Maternal mortality:**

    A. is 10 times higher following elective Caesarean section than after vaginal delivery
    B. is 6 times higher following emergency Caesarean section than after vaginal delivery

107. **An elective Caesarean section:**

    A. is essential for a woman who has had two previous Caesarean sections
    B. for breech presentation is associated with a higher level of maternal morbidity and mortality compared with vaginal delivery

108. The following relate to congenital abnormalities:

A. exomphalos occurs in the region of the umbilicus
B. measurement of serum 17-hydroxyprogesterone is essential in diagnosing congenital adrenal hyperplasia
C. there is a covering membrane at the base of exomphalos
D. gastroschisis defect is almost always on the left of a normal umbilical cord insertion
E. gastroschisis is commoner in girls
F. low birth weight and prematurity are commoner in gastroschisis than exomphalos
G. gastroschisis is associated with about a 50% incidence of chromosomal anomalies

109. External cephalic version:

A. at term may reduce the incidence of operative delivery
B. using tocolytic agents reduces complications
C. should always be performed in theatre
D. under ultrasound guidance is associated with lower complication rates
E. has a common complication of fetal death

110. With regard to endometrial resection:

A. danazol is the drug of choice preoperatively
B. laparoscopic sterilization is essential prior to the procedure
C. medical causes for menorrhagia should be excluded
D. it may take up to 4 months for the full effect to be judged
E. a xenon light source is superior to standard ones
F. postoperative bleeding would be an indication for laparotomy

111. **In epithelial ovarian cancer:**

    A. retroperitoneal lymph node spread is a late phenomenon
    B. the overall 5-year survival rate has changed very little over the years
    C. sodium thiosulphate is administered concurrently with intraperitoneal cisplatinum, with no increase in toxicity
    D. there is no role for cytotoxic chemotherapy

112. **Gonadotrophin-independent causes for precocious puberty include:**

    A. McCune–Albright syndrome
    B. premature thelarche
    C. primary hypothyroidism
    D. central precocious puberty

113. **In investigating infertility:**

    A. plasma progesterone of less than 20 nmol/l in the putative luteal phase is normal
    B. in a patient with regular cycles, serum prolactin is an essential investigation
    C. to save time for the couple, most investigations may be done in primary care
    D. a postcoital test assesses sperm function
    E. poor timing in the cycle is the common reason for a negative postcoital test
    F. luteinized unruptured follicle syndrome may be observed in women on indomethacin

114. **The following relate to hyperprolactinaemia:**

    A. it usually presents as primary amenorrhoea
    B. it may present as galactorrhoea
    C. it occurs in 70% of those who have given birth
    D. a CT scan may visualize 80% of microprolactinomas
    E. the condition may indicate subclinical hyperthyroidism

115. **With regard to ovarian hyperstimulation syndrome:**
    A. pericardial effusion is the commonest presentation
    B. it may occur if the corpora lutea are not stimulated
    C. serum E2 levels may predict development of the syndrome

116. **The following relate to the fallopian tubes:**
    A. 20% of the ampullary and fimbrial cells are ciliated
    B. the fertilized egg spends 6–8 days in the tube
    C. subsequent tubal occlusion occurs in about 36% of patients after two episodes of PID
    D. ascending PID infection predominantly affects the serosa
    E. isthmo–ampullary anastomoses are worse than isthmo–isthmic anastomoses of the tubes
    F. endometriosis is rarely associated with tubal pregnancy

117. **The following are unlikely causes of incontinence:**
    A. ectopic ureters
    B. bladder tumours
    C. interstitial cystitis
    D. depression
    E. antidepressants
    F. Parkinsonism
    G. fistula

118. **The following are true statements about sperm:**
    A. sperm production takes 3 to 4 weeks to complete
    B. sperm production is affected by a hot environment
    C. azoospermia indicates a low sperm count

119. The following relate to trophoblastic tumours:
    A. there is usually a unilateral adnexal mass
    B. they are associated with high titre beta hCG
    C. ultrasound features are pathognomonic
    D. they are more common in Africa
    E. there is no risk of recurrence in subsequent pregnancies
    F. the majority are malignant in young women

120. With regard to endometriosis:
    A. ovarian involvement is encountered in 25% of cases
    B. the incidence is increasing
    C. nasal mucosa may be involved
    D. a derivative of 17-alpha-ethinyl testosterone is used for treatment

121. Serum CA 125:
    A. is raised in about 35% of patients with ovarian cancer
    B. will differentiate between benign and malignant disease of the ovary
    C. is usually decreased in endometriosis
    D. is elevated in PID
    E. is of great value in premenopausal women

122. In a normal pregnancy:
    A. there is an increase in the peripheral vascular resistance
    B. cardiac output is halved
    C. uteroplacental circulation shows a low resistance

123. The following relate to laser treatment (light amplification by stimulated emission of radiation):
    A. Nd–YAG has the deepest penetration effect
    B. the CO_2 laser has the most shallow effect of all types of laser
    C. cutting and vaporization are obtained from the CO_2 laser
    D. penetration depth for the skin with the CO_2 laser is about 0.2 mm

124. Chronic pelvic pain is unlikely to be caused by:

A. Mittelschmerz syndrome
B. PCO
C. recurrent cystitis
D. Crohn's disease
E. diverticulitis
F. irritable bowel syndrome

125. Loss of vision in pregnancy may be due to:

A. pre-eclampsia and eclampsia
B. hyperemesis gravidarum
C. thrombotic disease
D. thrombotic thrombocytopenic purpura
E. migraine
F. optic neuritis
G. benign intracranial hypertension
H. pituitary adenoma
I. DIC

126. The following relate to D&C:

A. the procedure may overlook 1% of endometrial lesions
B. uterine perforation is around 1%
C. excessive bleeding occurs in the majority of patients

127. Mifepristone:

A. is an antioestrogen
B. is a derivative of norethisterone
C. has an antiglucocorticoid activity
D. is given intramuscularly
E. reaches a peak plasma concentration 4 hours after administration
F. may be used in medical terminations up to 15 weeks
G. may be used for cervical softening
H. may inhibit ovulation

128. **The following relate to chromosomal abnormalities:**
    A. the incidence is about 6 per 1000 births
    B. most Down's syndromes are due to meiotic-non-disjunction
    C. Edward's syndrome is a trisomy 13
    D. AFP levels are increased in most chromosomal diseases

129. **The following are true of ultrasound, when used to detect fetal abnormalities:**
    A. there is a high specificity with variable sensitivity
    B. NTD may be missed in about 30%
    C. cardiac abnormalities are usually easy to detect
    D. calyceal dilatation is usually an early development and may be detected early
    E. screening for neck abnormalities may reach 100%

130. **With regard to amniocentesis:**
    A. local anaesthetic is required
    B. it is safe to use methylene blue in cases of twins
    C. culture failure occurs in about 1–2%
    D. at 16 weeks the amniotic fluid volume is around 150–200 ml
    E. there is no role in late pregnancy

131. **The following are inherited as X-linked recessive:**
    A. haemophilia
    B. Tay–Sachs' disease
    C. beta thalassaemia
    D. Duchenne muscular dystrophy
    E. Lesch–Nyhan syndrome
    F. cystic fibrosis

132. The following are unlikely to cause urge syndrome:

    A. UTI
    B. interstitial cystitis
    C. pregnancy
    D. diabetes insipidus
    E. multiple sclerosis
    F. excessive fluid intake

133. The following are considered as contraindications for the use of Ventouse:

    A. face presentation
    B. active bleeding from fetal blood sample site
    C. prematurity
    D. fetal coagulation defect
    E. pregnancy complicated by sickle cell crisis

134. The following contraindicate vaginal hysterectomy:

    A. previous Caesarean section
    B. undiagnosed pelvic pain
    C. significant uterine enlargement
    D. previous uterine suspension
    E. invasive cervical lesions

135. The following relate to imperforate hymen:

    A. it typically occurs in 5–10-year-old girls
    B. dysmenorrhoea is common
    C. it may be associated with urinary retention
    D. secondary sexual development is usually absent

136. Endometriosis:

    A. may lead to infertility by causing ovulatory dysfunction
    B. if mild, often causes anatomical disruption
    C. may lead to infertility by causing abnormal fertilization
    D. may lead to infertility by causing early pregnancy loss
    E. is treated with danazol as the treatment of choice

137. **The following are ultrasound features of polycystic ovarian syndrome (PCO):**

    A. ten or more follicles, typically 2–8 mm in diameter
    B. central distribution of follicles
    C. decreased ovarian stroma
    D. diminished ovarian volume
    E. an enlarged uterus

138. **With regard to analgesia and anaesthesia during labour:**

    A. transmission of pain in the first stage of labour is related to the tenth, eleventh and twelfth thoracic and first lumbar spinal levels
    B. transmission of pain in the second stage of labour is related to the second to the fifth sacral spinal levels
    C. epidural analgesia is associated with hypertension
    D. blood patches are effective in treating spinal headache resulting from epidural analgesia
    E. epidural analgesia is known to affect the duration of the first stage of labour

139. **Childhood germ cell tumours include:**

    A. dysgerminoma
    B. yolk sac tumour
    C. immature teratoma
    D. embryonal carcinoma
    E. primary ovarian choriocarcinoma

140. **The following relate to the puerperium:**

    A. it only includes the first 4 weeks post-delivery
    B. 2 weeks after delivery, the uterus will have returned to the true pelvis
    C. beta human gonadotrophin will be negative 4 weeks after term delivery
    D. necrotizing fasciitis is a lethal complication that may result from perineal infection
    E. hypotension and ischaemic necrosis of the pituitary may result in panhypopituitarism (Sheehan's syndrome)
    F. in more than 80% of bottle-feeding mothers, the first period occurs by 6 weeks postpartum

141. The following relate to placental abruption:

   A. smoking is a contributory factor
   B. it is related to maternal age
   C. folic acid deficiency is a risk factor
   D. it is seen more frequently in cocaine users
   E. the risk of recurrence is 5–16%
   F. ultrasound is a useful tool for diagnosing the condition
   G. it is commoner in patients with renal transplants

142. The following are recognized complications of vacuum aspiration for termination of pregnancy:

   A. uterine perforation
   B. cervical laceration
   C. pelvic infection
   D. shock
   E. apnoea
   F. excessive haemorrhage
   G. maternal mortality of 1 in 10 000

143. With regard to the thyroid gland in pregnancy:

   A. there is a significant decrease in serum thyroxine-binding globulin
   B. if subtotal thyroidectomy is indicated, it is optimally performed in the second trimester
   C. mortality from neonatal thyrotoxicosis may be as high as 20%
   D. painful goitre and an increase in weight are common with transient postpartum hypothyroidism

144. The following are associated with smoking during pregnancy:

   A. ectopic pregnancy
   B. spontaneous miscarriage
   C. low birth weight
   D. sudden infant death syndrome
   E. eclampsia
   F. poor intellectual development in childhood
   G. placenta praevia
   H. impairment of physical growth

145. **A biophysical profile includes:**

    A. cardiotocography
    B. amniotic fluid volume
    C. fetal tone
    D. at least five gross fetal body movements
    E. continuous fetal breathing movements lasting for at least 1 minute
    F. ultrasound for 50 minutes

146. **The following relate to uterine inversion:**

    A. it is associated with fundal implantation of the placenta
    B. uterine hypotonia is not a risk factor
    C. if the placenta is still attached, it should be removed prior to replacement of the uterus
    D. the cervix remains open in the majority of cases
    E. it is commoner in Japanese women

147. **Endometrial hyperplasia:**

    A. is associated with heavy irregular menstruation
    B. is always due to exogenous hormonal stimulation
    C. usually resolves after D&C in women in the reproductive age group
    D. may be resolved by induction of ovulation
    E. is associated with endometrial cancer

148. **With regard to mixed mesodermal tumours of the uterus:**

    A. they are also known as carcinosarcomas
    B. they may contain smooth muscle elements
    C. they are common in old age
    D. exenteration is the treatment of choice for sarcoma botryoides
    E. pelvic irradiation may be a risk factor

149. **The following relate to gonadoblastomas:**

   A. they almost always occur in the gonads of intersexual patients
   B. the presence of a Y chromosome has been detected in over 90% of cases
   C. patients are usually phenotypically male
   D. the gonads should not be removed if the tumour is unilateral

150. **The following statements are correct:**

   A. mature cystic teratomas of the ovary are benign lesions
   B. the immature teratoma is derived only from mesoderm and endoderm
   C. Krukenberg tumours are usually bilateral
   D. 10% of cases of benign cystic teratoma are potentially malignant

151. **Obesity is associated with:**

   A. infertility
   B. ovarian cancer
   C. breast cancer
   D. polycystic ovaries
   E. urinary dysfunction
   F. IUGR

152. **Conservative management of ectopic pregnancy includes:**

   A. potassium iodide
   B. actinomycin
   C. mifepristone
   D. prostaglandins
   E. hyperosmolar glucose
   F. injection of methylene blue directly into the tube

153. The following may lead to premature ovarian failure:

    A. ataxia telangiectasia
    B. Down's syndrome
    C. Turner's syndrome
    D. DiGeorge syndrome
    E. pure gonadal dysgenesis
    F. iatrogenic causes
    G. excessive alcohol consumption

154. The following relate to ovarian tumours:

    A. serous adenocarcinomas comprise 90% of all malignant ovarian tumours
    B. psammoma bodies are characteristic features of serous adenocarcinoma
    C. at least one-third of serous adenocarcinomas are bilateral
    D. in endometrioid tumours, coexistent endometrial cancer is found in 20–30% of cases
    E. hobnail cells are characteristic features of mucinous tumours

155. The following are single-gene defects detectable by DNA amplification from single cells:

    A. sickle cell anaemia
    B. cystic fibrosis
    C. Duchenne muscular dystrophy
    D. Tay–Sachs' disease
    E. emphysema
    F. haemophilia A

156. The following are associated with early menarche:

    A. McCune–Albright syndrome
    B. adrenal oestrogen secreting tumours
    C. ovarian cysts
    D. brain trauma
    E. poverty

157. In polycystic ovarian syndrome:

   A. there is a raised FSH/LH ratio
   B. the patient frequently has a body mass index (BMI) of greater than 21
   C. the patient may present with hirsutism
   D. there is an increased risk of endometrial cancer
   E. if spontaneous pregnancy occurs, it is likely to be a multiple pregnancy
   F. levels of high density lipoprotein are usually elevated

158. The following relate to hyperemesis gravidarum:

   A. it is seen less frequently following a previous unsuccessful pregnancy
   B. the incidence is decreased in smokers
   C. it occurs less frequently in older women
   D. it is commonly seen in illegitimate pregnancies

159. The following medications may be used in the treatment of detrusor instability:

   A. doxepin
   B. salbutamol
   C. prazosin
   D. flunarizine
   E. imipramine
   F. medroxyprogesterone acetate

160. The features of congenital varicella syndrome include:

   A. microcephaly
   B. bilateral skin loss and skin scarring
   C. extra digits
   D. large-for-dates fetus
   E. chorioretinitis

161. **The following relate to genital tuberculosis:**

     A. it is almost always secondary
     B. the fallopian tubes are almost always involved
     C. menstrual disturbance occurs in about 70% of cases
     D. actinomycosis, sarcoidosis and histoplasmosis are all differential diagnoses
     E. infertility is the most common symptom
     F. mycobacteria are obligate anaerobes

162. **The following apply to normal bladder function:**

     A. urine enters the bladder at a rate of 5–10 ml per minute
     B. the first sensation of bladder filling is perceived at about 150–200 ml
     C. a strong desire to void is felt at about 500 ml
     D. baseline bladder pressure decreases during filling
     E. women require detrusor contraction to empty their bladders

163. **The following statements are correct:**

     A. insulin and insulin growth factor 1 both reduce the hepatic synthesis of sex hormones
     B. utilization of folic acid is increased by homocystinuria
     C. the incidence of postpartum haemorrhage (PPH) and neonatal jaundice is lower in prostaglandin induction of labour than in spontaneous labour

164. **The following relate to carcinomas of Bartholin's glands:**

     A. they account for 10–15% of all vulval cancers
     B. they are mostly adenocarcinomas and squamous carcinomas
     C. they may be transitional cell cancers
     D. 50% of patients will have lymph node metastases by the time of presentation
     E. they are commoner in black women

165. **With regard to clear cell adenocarcinoma:**

    A. it is seen predominantly in elderly women

    B. it is related to the use of diethylstilboestrol

    C. overall, the 5-year survival rate is about 30%

    D. hobnail cells are characteristic features

    E. abnormal vaginal smears are present in 20% of cases

166. **Adenomyosis:**

    A. affects young women

    B. and fibromyomas are co-associated in 40–50% of cases

    C. has primary dysmenorrhoea as the commonest presenting symptom

167. **The following relate to endometrial hyperplasia:**

    A. it results from prolonged unopposed oestrogen hyperstimulation of the ovary

    B. it occurs typically at the beginning and at the end of the reproductive era

    C. it occurs typically in obese, anovulating women

    D. LHRH analogue therapy is used in older women

    E. induction of ovulation is used to revert hyperplasia

    F. wedge resection is one of the methods used for treating hyperplasia

168. **The following are recognized causes of non-androgen-dependent hirsutism:**

    A. race

    B. pregnancy

    C. hypothyroidism

    D. cranial injury

    E. PCO

    F. acromegaly

169. **With regard to vaginal melanoma:**

    A. it is a common condition

    B. it commonly presents in the upper vagina

    C. surgical treatment is curative

170. **In pseudocyesis:**

   A. both symptoms and signs of pregnancy may be obvious
   B. there is an element of fear of getting pregnant

171. **Virilism is associated with:**

   A. endometrial tumours
   B. 5-alpha-reductase deficiency
   C. absent mullerian factor
   D. true hermaphroditism
   E. adrenal hyperplasia

172. **With regard to blood:**

   A. HbA is composed of a pair of alpha and a pair of beta chains
   B. fetal haemoglobin accounts for less than 1% of the haemoglobin in adults
   C. the alpha chains of the fetal haemoglobin are replaced by gamma chains
   D. sickle cell syndrome is an autosomal inherited disorder
   E. the risk of sickle cell crisis increases during pregnancy
   F. the homozygous form of alpha thalassaemia is not compatible with life
   G. Hodgkin's disease is affected by pregnancy

173. **The following relate to thrombocytopenia in pregnant women:**

   A. it may be secondary to SLE
   B. it rarely affects the fetus
   C. splenectomy is a safe treatment later in pregnancy
   D. Caesarean section is indicated in the majority of patients

174. **Fragile X syndrome:**

   A. is a common cause of mental retardation
   B. commonly affects females
   C. often gives a false negative result with amniocentesis

175. **The following relate to Von Willebrand's disease:**

A. there is deficiency of factor VIII
B. there is a defect in platelet function
C. it is an autosomal recessive condition
D. cryoprecipitate can be used as a method of treatment
E. secondary postpartum haemorrhage is a recognized complication
F. menorrhagia is a contraindication for the use of the combined oral contraceptive pill

176. **With regard to the menopause:**

A. venous disease is the major cause of death in the postmenopausal woman
B. psychological complaints affect between 25 and 50% of women during the menopause
C. urethral syndrome during the menopause is mainly due to lack of oestrogen
D. bone loss accelerates in the first 2 years following the menopause
E. the development of osteoporosis is determined by peak bone mass and the rate of bone loss
F. the onset of the menopause is related to socio-economic factors, race, weight and height of the patient
G. levels of oestradiol and androstenedione secreted by the ovaries are unchanged

177. **Vasomotor symptoms of the menopause include:**

A. palpitations
B. sweats
C. hot flushes
D. poor memory
E. insomnia
F. irritability
G. anorgasmia

178. **Secondary osteoporosis is associated with the following conditions:**

    A. diabetes mellitus
    B. hypoparathyroidism
    C. anticonvulsant therapy
    D. gastrectomy
    E. malabsorption syndrome
    F. chronic neurological disease
    G. chronic obstructive airways disease
    H. malignancy
    I. hypogonadism

179. **The following are recognized causes of urinary incontinence:**

    A. overflow incontinence
    B. congenital causes
    C. urethral diverticulae
    D. urinary tract infection
    E. faecal impaction
    F. immobility

180. **The symptoms of urogenital atrophy include:**

    A. vaginal moistening
    B. pruritis
    C. dysmenorrhoea
    D. prolapse
    E. urgency, frequency, dysuria and urinary tract infections

181. **Tibolone:**

    A. is a synthetic steroid compound
    B. has strong oestrogenic and progestogenic properties
    C. has very weak androgenic properties
    D. has a high incidence of withdrawal bleeding
    E. is suitable for long-term use in the postmenopausal woman
    F. is indicated for the perimenopausal woman who is still menstruating
    G. metabolism takes place in the liver and the intestine
    H. suppresses FSH and to a lesser extent LH

182. The following relate to spermicides:

   A. spermicides on their own are effective contraceptive methods

   B. the most commonly used spermicide in Britain is nonoxynol-8

   C. most spermicides have a rapid antimicrobial effect against Chlamydia

   D. usage of spermicides may lead to vaginal ulceration

183. In grade 3 (severe) ovarian hyperstimulation syndrome:

   A. the symptoms include pronounced abdominal distension and pain

   B. pleural effusion may occur

   C. hospitalization is not necessary for treatment

   D. symptoms may be prolonged if conception has occurred

   E. extrauterine pregnancy is unlikely to result in the condition

   F. this is a particular risk for women with polycystic ovaries

184. The following relate to hyperprolactinaemia:

   A. it is a known cause of ovulatory dysfunction

   B. it is unlikely to be due to a space-occupying lesion

   C. when hyperprolactinaemia is suspected, further tests to exclude hyperthyroidism are indicated

   D. dopamine antagonists can be used to treat hyperprolactinaemia

185. The following may cause secondary amenorrhoea:

   A. polycystic ovary syndrome

   B. premature ovarian failure

   C. hypoprolactinaemia

   D. severe weight loss

   E. severe weight gain

   F. hypergonadotrophic hypogonadism

186. **Oocyte donation is indicated in the following:**

    A. genetic disease carrier status
    B. failed IVF
    C. habitual miscarriage
    D. gonadal dysgenesis
    E. premature ovarian failure

187. **With regard to phaeochromocytoma:**

    A. it arises from the adrenal cortex
    B. it produces excessive catecholamines
    C. stress may provoke symptoms of phaeochromocytoma
    D. surgical removal of the tumour in early pregnancy has no effect on the outcome of the pregnancy
    E. in a patient with phaeochromocytoma, there is no contraindication for vaginal delivery
    F. it may be a familial tumour

188. **The following relate to endocervical adenocarcinoma:**

    A. a barrel-shaped cervix is a characteristic feature
    B. it is increasing in incidence
    C. the incidence is decreasing in young women

189. **The following are differential diagnoses for hyperemesis gravidarum:**

    A. thyrotoxicosis
    B. hypoparathyroidism
    C. diabetic ketoacidosis
    D. appendicitis
    E. pancreatitis
    F. pyelonephritis
    G. large bowel obstruction

190. **The following relate to Stamey endoscopic bladder neck suspension:**

   A. it has an important role in managing complex cases of stress incontinence
   B. it is indicated mainly for young patients
   C. the procedure is contraindicated in a patient who has had multiple unsuccessful operations

191. **With regard to anticoagulants in pregnancy:**

   A. chondrodysplasia punctata is associated with heparin usage
   B. nasal deformity is caused by warfarin
   C. diaphragmatic hernia has an association with warfarin therapy
   D. teratogenic effects due to warfarin are limited to the first trimester
   E. microcephaly is associated with heparin usage
   F. heparin is linked to bone demineralization in the fetus

192. **The following relate to cardiac disease in pregnancy:**

   A. cyanosis is only seen with pulmonary stenosis
   B. in pulmonary stenosis, heart failure depends on the degree of stenosis
   C. patent ductus arteriosus results in a permanent reversed shunt
   D. atrial septal defect may give rise to a shunt from the left to the right side of the heart
   E. in Eisenmenger's complex, interventricular septal defect is rarely seen
   F. cyanosis is an early feature in Eisenmenger's complex
   G. should Caesarean section be required in patients with heart disease, spinal anaesthesia should be avoided

193. **The following are known complications of endometrial resection:**

    A. perforation of the uterus
    B. excessive haemorrhage
    C. circulatory overload
    D. anaphylactic haemolytic anaemia

194. **The combined oral contraceptive pill has the following benefits:**

    A. the incidence of ovarian cancer is reduced by 10%
    B. the incidence of endometrial cancer is reduced by 5–10%
    C. there is a reduction in the incidence of potentially malignant breast disease
    D. there is a reduction in the incidence of uterine fibroids by about 50%
    E. the incidence of pelvic inflammatory disease is increased by 30%

195. **The following relate to antihypertensives in pregnancy:**

    A. neonates born to mothers who were given methyldopa show an increase in head circumference
    B. diuretics are linked with neonatal thrombocytopenia
    C. atenolol is contraindicated in pregnancy
    D. captopril in pregnancy is associated with congenital renal agenesis

196. **The following are recognized effects of combined oral contraceptive pills:**

    A. they stimulate the synthesis of transport proteins in the liver
    B. there is an increased blood level of thyroxine-binding globulin
    C. there is a reduction in sex-hormone-binding globulin
    D. total plasma concentration of sex-hormone-binding globulin is increased
    E. most clotting factors are decreased

197. With regard to the exenteration procedure:

A. current carcinoma of the cervix is the main indication for the exenteration procedure

B. exenteration may be performed if there is evidence of spread of the tumour outside the pelvis

C. in anterior exenteration, the rectum is preserved

D. should small bowel obstruction occur following exenteration, it should be treated surgically

E. survival rate varies from 50 to 80%

198. Danazol:

A. is an isoxazol derivative of 19-alpha-ethinyl testosterone

B. indirectly inhibits ovarian and adrenal steroidogenesis

C. causes a low level of oestrogen and atrophy of the endometrium during its use

D. has side-effects that are dose dependent

199. The following relate to mature cystic teratoma (dermoid cyst):

A. it is an epithelial cell tumour

B. it is usually formed from fully mature elements

C. the presence of hair is a characteristic feature

D. well-formed teeth occur in 70% of cases

E. a mature cystic teratoma of the ovary behaves like that of the testis

200. In statistics:

A. the birth rate is the number of births in one year multiplied by 1000 and divided by the mid-year population

B. the fertility rate is the number of births in one year multiplied by 1000 and divided by the number of women aged 15–44 years

C. maternal mortality rates are expressed by relating the number of maternal deaths to births occurring in the same period of time

D. the perinatal mortality rate is the number of perinatal deaths, stillbirths after 24 weeks and first-week neonatal deaths expressed as a proportion of 1000 births occurring in the same area at the same time

201. The following are predominant features of haematocolpos:

    A. dysmenorrhoea
    B. abdominal pain
    C. interference with defaecation

202. In Klinefelter's syndrome:

    A. the chromosomal pattern is 46XXY
    B. the patient usually has microtestes
    C. gynaecomastia is an unlikely presentation

203. The following relate to ovarian steroidogenesis:

    A. the hormone LH promotes ovarian steroidogenesis
    B. the ovarian stroma synthesizes androstenedione
    C. oestradiol is synthesized mainly by the follicles
    D. progesterone is the dominant hormone produced by the corpus luteum

204. With regard to Laurence–Moon–Biedl syndrome:

    A. retinitis pigmentosa is a classical feature of the syndrome
    B. polydactyly is a recognized feature
    C. syndactyly is rarely identified
    D. mental retardation will be evident later in life

205. Virilism is defined by one or more of the following features:

    A. clitoral hypertrophy
    B. breast hypertrophy
    C. male type baldness
    D. deepening of the voice

206. The following relate to the human placenta:

    A. hormone, steroid and protein production are known functions of the placenta

    B. active transport is a recognized phenomenon

    C. simple diffusion is not a recognized function

    D. pinocytosis is a recognized phenomenon

    E. leakage is a special process attributed to the human placenta

207. The following are biological roles of relaxin in mammals:

    A. stimulation of myometrial activity during pregnancy

    B. cervical ripening

    C. mammary growth during pregnancy

    D. inhibition of sperm mobility

208. The following are identifiable predisposing factors in hypertensive disorders of pregnancy:

    A. age

    B. parity

    C. partner's blood group

    D. obesity

    E. smoking

    F. family history

209. The following relate to alpha thalassaemia:

    A. it is common in South East Asia

    B. beta-chain synthesis is suppressed

    C. the homozygous form is compatible with life

210. With regard to Hodgkin's disease in pregnancy:

    A. the course of Hodgkin's disease is usually affected by pregnancy

    B. should pregnancy occur in a patient with Hodgkin's disease, it is usually complicated

    C. pregnancy in a patient with Hodgkin's disease should be terminated early

    D. treatment of advanced Hodgkin's disease in pregnancy should be surgery followed by radiotherapy

211. **Ritodrine hydrochloride:**
    A. is contraindicated in cases of eclampsia
    B. can be used safely in cases of chorioamnionitis
    C. can be used in the first or second trimesters
    D. may cause hyperkalaemia
    E. may cause salivary gland enlargement
    F. may cause agranulocytosis
    G. can be used with caution in patients with cardiac disease

212. **The following relate to urinary calculus in pregnancy:**
    A. the incidence is between 5 and 10% of all pregnancies
    B. calcium oxalate or phosphate is commonly seen in patients with calculus disease in pregnancy
    C. infections with calculi are commonly caused by *Proteus mirabilis*
    D. suppression of fetal parathormone levels is a recognized feature in pregnant women with calculus disease in pregnancy

213. **With regard to eclampsia:**
    A. diazepam, when given to halt seizures, does not affect the fetal heart beat
    B. chlormethiazole, when used in eclampsia, carries a risk of maternal respiratory depression and fluid overload
    C. chlormethiazole is a sedative drug
    D. use of magnesium sulphate may lead to hypercalcaemia

214. The following are true statements about Down's syndrome:

A. the incidence is about 1 in 200 pregnancies
B. the majority of cases are the result of trisomy 21
C. should translocation occur, it is usually between chromosomes 14 and 21
D. the majority of Down's cases will be found to have an IQ of less than 50 when they are 10 years old
E. the incidence of Alzheimer's disease in Down's syndrome is higher than in the general population
F. heart problems occur in 10% of cases of Down's syndrome
G. two-thirds of Down's syndrome babies are born to women who are less than 35 years old

215. The following relate to chorioamnionitis:

A. the diagnosis is based on the histological finding of polymorphonuclear leukocyte infiltration
B. it is associated with recovery of bacteria in about 70% of cases
C. the incidence of chorioamnionitis is lower in women delivering preterm rather than term babies
D. it may lead to sepsis and death in utero

216. The following are possible causes of tubal disease associated with infertility:

A. pelvic inflammatory disease
B. endometriosis
C. previous abdominal or pelvic surgery
D. previous history of ectopic pregnancy
E. segmental atresia of the tube
F. excessive convolution of the tube

217. In a normal pregnancy:

A. there is an increase in the peripheral vascular resistance
B. there is an increased plasma volume
C. there is a decreased cardiac output
D. there is an enlargement of the heart

218. **With regard to peptic ulcer in pregnancy:**

   A. peptic ulcer is common in pregnancy
   B. it is related to female sex hormones
   C. it should be suspected if there is severe epigastric pain showing nocturnal exacerbation

219. **The following relate to gonorrhoea in pregnancy:**

   A. it is almost always symptomatic
   B. it may present as acute urethritis
   C. it may present with excessive vaginal discharge
   D. it may present with abdominal pain
   E. rectal and urethral swabs should always be performed
   F. amoxycillin 3 g may be given orally as a single dose for treating the condition in pregnancy

220. **The following drugs should be avoided if possible during breast feeding:**

   A. metranidozole
   B. augmentin
   C. tetracycline
   D. sulfonamide
   E. choramphenicol

221. **The following relate to intestinal infestations in pregnancy:**

   A. *Taenia saginata* and *Taenia solium* are likely to cause problems in pregnancy
   B. niclosamide should be used as a single dose in pregnancy
   C. dichlorophen may be used in pregnancy
   D. *Ascaris lumbricoides* should only be treated when the infection is severe
   E. *Enterobius vermicularis* has no serious side effects in pregnancy
   F. anaemia may result from hookworm infestation
   G. metranidazole (Flagyl) may be used in pregnancy

222. **The following factors are known to affect the interpretation of serum marker results:**
    A. multiple pregnancy
    B. missed abortion
    C. race
    D. insulin-dependent diabetes mellitus
    E. repeat testing

223. **Concerning the frequency of structural anomalies:**
    A. the incidence of craniospinal anomalies is 10 per 1000 births
    B. the incidence of cardiovascular anomalies is 1–2 per 1000 births
    C. the incidence of severe renal tract anomalies is 1 per 1000 births
    D. the incidence of gastrointestinal anomalies is 1 per 100 births

224. **Fetal tissue sampling could help prenatal diagnoses in the following conditions:**
    A. neuro-axonal degeneration
    B. epidermolytic hyperkeratosis
    C. epidermolysis bullosa dystrophica
    D. contact dermatitis

225. **The following relate to obstetric haemorrhage:**
    A. the risk of death from this condition is about 1 in 10 000 deliveries in the UK
    B. primary postpartum haemorrhage may occur after 5% of deliveries
    C. ligation of the internal iliac artery prevents hysterectomy in 90% of obstetric haemorrhages

226. The following relate to double and ectopic ureters:

    A. complete or partial duplication of the ureter results from late splitting of the ureteric bud

    B. with double ureters, the kidneys usually completely separate

    C. an ectopic ureter may open into the trigone

    D. ectopic ureters opening below the urethral sphincter do not usually give any clinical or anatomical symptoms

227. The following apply to sling operations for urinary incontinence:

    A. suburethral slings are usually reserved for cases of recurrent stress incontinence

    B. strips of rectus fascia or external oblique fascia are commonly used

    C. a combined abdominal and vaginal approach is not necessary

228. The following relate to fistulae:

    A. vesicogenital tract fistulae are most likely after colporrhaphy and vaginal and abdominal hysterectomy

    B. bladder neck fistulae are the most simple fistulae to treat

    C. the fistulae between the urinary and the genital tracts characteristically present with continuous leakage of urine

    D. most vesicovaginal fistulae can be closed through the vaginal route

229. The following are recognized predisposing factors for puerperal sepsis:

    A. prolonged ruptured membranes

    B. prolonged labour

    C. operative delivery

    D. history of pelvic sepsis

230. With regard to cancer of the cervix:

A. the overall survival in stage 1 disease is about 40%
B. the survival rate is about 90% in node-negative patients
C. the size of the tumour is related to survival rate
D. early recurrence of cervical cancer has no association with mortality

231. In testicular feminization syndrome:

A. the patient may appear to be a normal female
B. the patient usually has testes and is genotypically XY
C. the incidence is 1 in 10 000
D. the condition is sex-linked recessive

232. The following relate to fibroids:

A. pressure symptoms involve urinary and bowel functions
B. sarcomatous change occurs in more than 10%
C. polycythaemia is due to secretion of a erythopoeitin-like substance
D. intramural fibroids are fibroids within the uterine wall, surrounded by a true capsule
E. intraligamentary fibroids grow within the broad ligament and can cause ureteric compression
F. fibroids are composed of striated muscle cells

233. The following are unlikely causes of hirsutism:

A. hyperthecosis of the ovary
B. thyroid disease
C. acromegaly
D. anorexia nervosa
E. Turner's syndrome

234. The following drugs may cause hypoprolactinaemia:

A. cimetidine
B. opiates
C. prochlorperazine

235. **The following relate to pseudomyxoma peritonei:**

    A. it is a benign mucinous tumour of the ovary
    B. the tumour is of intestinal type
    C. it may lead to bowel obstruction
    D. repeat evacuation of mucin may be indicated

236. **Sarcoma botryoides:**

    A. is a low grade, malignant tumour
    B. commonly occurs after the age of 10 years
    C. may be diagnosed on abdominal examination
    D. may be treated by chemotherapy

237. **The following could be considered in the differential diagnosis of premenstrual syndrome:**

    A. endometriosis
    B. hypothyroidism
    C. the menopause
    D. psychosexual problems

238. **The following are contraindications for epidural analgesia:**

    A. maternal refusal
    B. evident coagulopathy
    C. severe thrombocytopenia
    D. generalized or localized sepsis

239. **The following are unlikely in the aetiology of hydrops fetalis:**

    A. diaphragmatic hernia
    B. posterior urethral valves
    C. umbilical cord thrombosis
    D. chorioangioma
    E. beta thalassaemia
    F. G6PD deficiency

240. The following relate to Arias–Stella reaction:

    A. the nuclear sizes are usually the same
    B. there is nuclear hypertrophy
    C. the quantity of cytoplasm is reduced
    D. it is likely to be mistaken for endometriosis

241. With regard to abdominal ectopic pregnancy:

    A. the incidence is 1 in 8000 to 10 000
    B. it is common in young patients
    C. the incidence is directly related to parity
    D. when diagnosed, endometriosis is frequently reported
    E. the placenta must be removed in all cases

242. The following infections are dangerous to the fetus and newborn child:

    A. herpes simplex
    B. measles
    C. coxsackievirus
    D. influenza

243. Abnormal lactation may be due to:

    A. choriocarcinoma
    B. corpus luteum cysts
    C. oestrogen-secreting adrenal tumours

244. The following are recognized features of congenital rubella infection

    A. patent ductus arteriosus
    B. hydrocephalus
    C. thrombocytopenia
    D. interstitial pneumonia

245. The following are causes of neonatal seizures:

    A. hypercalcaemia
    B. water intoxication
    C. hypernatraemia
    D. rubella encephalitis
    E. narcotic withdrawal
    F. congenital toxoplasmosis

246. The following relate to human chorionic gonadotrophin (hCG):

A. it is a glycoprotein
B. it has the action of the pituitary luteinizing hormone
C. in first trimester abortion, a minimum of 37 days is needed before beta human chorionic gonadotrophin is negative

247. The normal vaginal flora includes:

A. Clostridia
B. Enterococcus
C. aerobic streptococci
D. Listeria species

248. Erythromycin:

A. acts mainly against gram-negative organisms
B. is related to macrolides
C. activity is enhanced at acidic pH
D. acts by inhibiting protein synthesis
E. can be given intravenously

249. With regard to herpes gestationis:

A. it is an autoimmune disease
B. it may be caused by herpes virus
C. it develops in the first trimester
D. maternal prognosis is excellent
E. spontaneous cure is expected in 40%

250. The following are classified as spirochaetes:

A. Borrelia
B. Leptospira
C. Yaws virus

251. The following statements are true:

A. in the gynaecoid pelvis, the interspinous diameter is shortened
B. the pubic arch is usually curved in the android pelvis
C. the inclination of the sacrum is usually anteriorly in the android pelvis

252. **The following relate to phaeochromocytoma:**

    A. the ovary is a known ectopic site
    B. it is common during pregnancy
    C. about 40% of tumours are benign in adults
    D. alpha adrenergic agents are the treatment of choice

253. **With regard to rooming-in:**

    A. the chances of the infant contracting infections are increased
    B. it is usually expensive

254. **The following relate to prolapsed umbilical cord:**

    A. the incidence of occult prolapse is 1 in 20
    B. it may be due to cephalopelvic disproportion
    C. it results from a short cord of less than 20 cm

255. **In acute fatty liver of pregnancy:**

    A. haemoptysis is a typical feature
    B. viral hepatitis is a known differential diagnosis
    C. malnutrition may be the cause
    D. maternal mortality is about 20%
    E. it is commoner in Europeans

256. **With regard to myasthenia gravis:**

    A. pregnancy causes relapses even during the early weeks
    B. the most critical time is the first trimester
    C. there is no effect of myasthenia gravis on pregnancy
    D. scopolamine is safe in a pregnant patient with myasthenia gravis
    E. transient neonatal myasthenia gravis is seen in 2%

257. **The following relate to ovarian pregnancy:**

    A. it may be diagnosed clinically
    B. a positive pregnancy test is common
    C. ovarian rupture is likely in 30%
    D. hysterectomy is usually indicated

258. **The following conditions are unlikely to be detected antenatally:**

    A. cri du chat syndrome
    B. Gaucher's disease
    C. Niemann–Pick disease type A
    D. colour of eyes
    E. cystinuria
    F. congenital nephrosis
    G. xeroderma pigmentosum

259. **Fetal tachycardia may be due to:**

    A. extreme prematurity
    B. maternal hypothyroidism
    C. fetal hypervolaemia
    D. chorioamnionitis
    E. maternal hyperthermia

260. **The following are examples of X-linked recessive conditions and traits:**

    A. haemophilia A
    B. haemophilia B
    C. gonadal dysgenesis, XY type
    D. cervico-oculo-acoustic syndrome
    E. Marfan's syndrome
    F. Huntington's chorea
    G. night blindness

261. **With regard to anorexia nervosa:**

    A. levels of serum LH are high
    B. hirsutism often occurs
    C. young patients have a good outcome

262. **The soft chancre (chancroid):**

    A. is a venereal disease
    B. is caused by gram-positive rods
    C. is characterized by a painless genital ulcer
    D. is characterized by a long incubation period

263. **The following relate to sarcoma of the cervix:**

   A. it arises from the mullerian duct
   B. it is common in a young age group (20–30 years)
   C. there is a known association with sexual behaviour
   D. it frequently metastasizes to the lung

ANSWERS

1. A. False
   B. True
   C. True
   D. True
   E. False

The incidence of placenta praevia increases with parity and is commoner in women who have had previous surgery. It is associated with IUGR, possibly because of poor placentation.

2. A. True
   B. True
   C. False
   D. True
   E. True
   F. True
   G. False
   H. True
   I. True

3. A. False
   B. False
   C. False
   D. False
   E. False

A–E are all known contraindications to the use of COCs.

4. A. True
   B. False
   C. True
   D. True
   E. True

Placenta accreta refers to a placenta that is abnormally adherent to the uterine muscle and is characterized by paucity of the underlying decidua. Any condition leading to reduction of the decidua can lead to abnormal adherence, e.g. previous infection, uterine scar or previous traumatic curettage.

5.   A. True
     B. False
     C. False
     D. True

Thecomas are more common in women in their 50s and 60s.

6.   A. False
     B. True
     C. True
     D. True
     E. False
     F. False

7.   A. True
     B. True
     C. True
     D. True
     E. False

8.   A. True
     B. False
     C. False
     D. True
     E. True
     F. False

Cis platin is given intravenously and can cause
hypomagnesaemia. It is nephrotoxic and pretreatment
hydration is mandatory.

9.   A. True
     B. False
     C. False
     D. True
     E. False

Transmission of cytomegalovirus infection to the fetus may
occur in any trimester, but is severe in early or late pregnancy.

10. A. **False**
     B. **True**
     C. **False**

Benign physiological ovarian cysts are not uncommon in the first trimester and most are no longer present by 16 weeks' gestation. Laparotomy is advisable in the second trimester in the majority of cases. Approximately 4% of ovarian tumours diagnosed in pregnancy are malignant.

11. A. **True**
     B. **True**
     C. **False**
     D. **True**
     E. **True**

12. A. **True**
     B. **True**
     C. **True**

13. A. **False**
     B. **True**
     C. **False**
     D. **False**
     E. **False**

There is no significant association between fallopian tube tumours and ectopic pregnancies. Metastatic tumours from colonic carcinoma are sometimes found. The 5-year survival for fallopian tube cancer is 25–35% and profuse vaginal discharge is the commonest presentation.

14. A. **False**
     B. **True**
     C. **True**
     D. **False**
     E. **True**

The amnion is only a single cell layer and is of fetal ectodermal origin. Human chorionic gonadotrophin is produced by the syncytiotrophoblast.

15. A. True
    B. True
    C. True
    D. True
    E. True
    F. False

16. A. True
    B. True
    C. False
    D. False
    E. False
    F. False

17. A. True
    B. False

Papillomaviruses are double-stranded DNA viruses.

18. A. True
    B. False
    C. True
    D. False

A single umbilical artery is found in 1% of singleton pregnancies and 7% of multiple pregnancies. It has an association with genitourinary, cardiovascular, orofacial and musculoskeletal abnormalities.

19. A. False
    B. True
    C. False

The majority of transverse vaginal septa occur at the junction of the middle and upper two-thirds of the vagina. Williams' vulvovaginoplasty is an operation for the absence of vagina.

20. A. False
    B. True
    C. True
    D. True
    E. True
    F. True

21. A. False
    B. False
    C. True
    D. False

Rapid cytogenic results may be obtained within 12–24 hours. Fetal loss occurs in 1.8–4.5%. There is a 1–1.5% incidence of confined placenta or pseudo-mosaicism, where a discrepancy exists between chorionic and fetal karyotypes.

22. A. True
    B. False
    C. True
    D. True
    E. False

Hypoplasia, not hyperplasia, should be considered in postmature pregnancy.

23. A. False
    B. True
    C. True
    D. True
    E. False
    F. True
    G. True
    H. False
    I. False
    J. True

The herpes virus is a double-stranded DNA virus.

24. A. True
    B. True
    C. True
    D. False
    E. True
    F. False
    G. True
    H. False
    I. False
    J. False

A woman who is HIV positive has a 50% chance of developing AIDS in 5 years.

25. A. False
    B. True
    C. False
    D. True
    E. True

26. A. True
    B. False
    C. True
    D. False

There are fewer than 1 × 106/ml white blood cells in a normal semen analysis. There is at least 2.4 μmol of zinc per ejaculate, not calcium.

27. A. True
    B. False
    C. False
    D. True
    E. False
    F. False
    G. False
    H. True
    I. True
    J. False

Trichomonads are unicellular organisms. Clue cells are diagnostic of bacterial vaginosis. *Trichomonas vaginalis* is not generally a cause of systemic disease.

28. A. False
     B. True
     C. True
     D. False

29. A. False
     B. False
     C. False
     D. True
     E. True
     F. False
     G. False

The condition is unlikely in pregnancy or following sterilization. Infection rarely occurs in midcycle.

30. A. True
     B. False
     C. False
     D. True

Diabetes mellitus, not diabetes insipidus, is associated with fetal macrosomia.

31. A. True
     B. False
     C. True
     D. False
     E. False

A short sternum is a feature in Edward's syndrome.

32. A. True
     B. False
     C. True
     D. False
     E. False

Spermatogenesis is affected by hyperthermia, not hypothermia.

33. A. True
    B. False
    C. True
    D. False
    E. False

At term, the volume of amniotic fluid is 800–900 ml. Infantile polycystic kidneys and cord compression are both associated with oligohydramnios, not polyhydramnios.

34. A. False
    B. True
    C. True
    D. True

35. A. True
    B. False
    C. False
    D. False

There is an increased incidence of both abruption and placenta praevia in multiple pregnancy. Cephalic/cephalic presentation occurs in about 40%. If the pregnancy is progressing with no complications, interference is not advisable.

36. A. False
    B. True
    C. True
    D. False
    E. False

Dysgerminoma is a sex cord stromal tumour and gonadoblastoma is a germ cell tumour.

37. A. True
    B. True
    C. False

Anaemia is associated with asymmetrical IUGR.

38. A. False
B. True
C. False
D. False

RU486 produces changes in the histology of the endometrium.

39. A. False
B. True
C. False
D. True
E. True

Abruptio placenta is a complication of cocaine during pregnancy, not placenta praevia.

40. A. True
B. True
C. True
D. False

41. A. True
B. True
C. False
D. False

Encephalopathy, not encephalitis, is associated with hyperemesis gravidarum. There is no evidence that the condition is commoner in IVF compared to spontaneous pregnancies.

42. A. True
B. False
C. False
D. True
E. False

Hypoglycaemia, hypocalcaemia and hyperbilirubinaemia are known neonatal complications.

43. A. True
    B. False
    C. True
    D. False
    E. False

Implants are effective for 5 years, are suitable for obese women and cause menstrual abnormalities in about 60% of users.

44. A. True
    B. False
    C. True
    D. False

Depending on the population, the incidence of gestational diabetes varies. This figure is what is expected from European data. Diet control may be enough in some cases. With reasonable control, there is no need to interfere before 40 weeks.

45. A. False
    B. True
    C. False
    D. True
    E. True

Ovulation occurs approximately 10–12 hours after the LH peak. The LH peak occurs 34–36 hours before follicular rupture.

46. A. False
    B. False

The incubation period for rubella is 14–21 days.

47. A. True
    B. False
    C. False
    D. False
    E. True

The perforation rate varies between 0.6 and 1.3 per 1000 insertions (WHO 1987).

48.   A. False
      B. False
      C. False
      D. False

A–D are all associated with high blood pressure in early pregnancy.

49.   A. True
      B. False
      C. False
      D. True
      E. True
      F. False
      G. True

In the complete hydatidiform mole, all chromosomes are paternally derived and the commonest chromosome is 46XX. There is a 15–20% malignant potential for the complete mole.

50.   A. True
      B. False
      C. False
      D. False

51.   A. True
      B. True
      C. False
      D. True
      E. True

The bladder has a transitional cell lining, not squamous cell.

52.   A. False
      B. False
      C. False
      D. False

Sheehan's syndrome results from postpartum haemorrhage. It may lead to panhypopituitarism with the onset of symptoms occurring usually during the postpartum period. There is lack of lactation because of decreased prolactin and this is usually the first recognized pituitary deficiency. There are symptoms of hypothyroidism, hypoadrenalism and hypogonadotropism, which usually become evident later.

53. A. False
     B. True
     C. True
     D. False
     E. False

Serum hCG is usually low in placental site trophoblastic
tumours. Villi are characteristically absent and there is a high
serum placental lactogen.

54. A. True
     B. True
     C. True
     D. False
     E. False
     F. True
     G. False

Coarctation of the aorta, not aortic incompetence, is a feature
of Turner's syndrome. The oestrogen level is low.

55. A. True
     B. True
     C. False
     D. False
     E. False

It is azoospermia, not oligospermia, that is a characteristic
feature. Testicular volume rarely exceeds 4 ml and the prostate
is usually small.

56. A. False
     B. True
     C. True
     D. True
     E. False
     F. True

There is usually no bacteriuria associated with the syndrome.
Symptoms occasionally relate to the menstrual cycle.

57. A. False
    B. False
    C. False
    D. True
    E. True

The diaphragm is available in sizes from 55 to 100 mm. It can be inserted at any time during intercourse and should remain in place for at least 6 hours after intercourse.

58. A. True
    B. True
    C. False
    D. False
    E. False

Malignant changes are seen very rarely (0.3–0.7% of cases).

59. A. False
    B. True
    C. True
    D. True
    E. True
    F. False
    G. True
    H. True
    I. True

60. A. False
    B. True
    C. False

Childbirth has a curative effect on primary dysmenorrhoea. In pelvic inflammatory disease, the pain usually occurs in the few days following menstruation.

61. A. True
    B. True
    C. True
    D. False
    E. True

The failure rate depends of the stage of the menstrual cycle.

62. A. True
B. True
C. True
D. True
E. True

63. A. True
B. True
C. False
D. False
E. False

64. A. False
B. True
C. True
D. False
E. False

65. A. False
B. True
C. True
D. True
E. True
F. False
G. False

66. A. False
B. True
C. False

Most women with menorrhagia will have normal haemoglobin levels.

67. A. False
B. False
C. False
D. True
E. False

Hinselmann introduced colposcopy in 1925. Iodine will identify areas that are glycogen deficient. Colposcopy is not a method of screening for cervical cancer.

68. **A.** False
     B. True
     C. False
     D. False

Secretion has no relation to menstruation. The common rule 'always drain the abscess' should be followed.

69. **A.** True
     B. False
     C. False
     D. True

70. **A.** True
     B. True
     C. False
     D. False
     E. True
     F. False
     G. False
     H. True
     I. True
     J. False
     K. True
     L. True
     M. True

The lesion is usually thin. Involvement of trunk and limbs may occur in up to 18% of patients. It is epidermal atrophy, not hypertrophy, that is a characteristic feature.

71. **A.** False
     B. True
     C. True
     D. False
     E. True

72. **A.** True
     B. False
     C. False
     D. False

The aetiology of NTDs is multifactorial. The recurrence is about 1%.

73. A. True
    B. True
    C. True
    D. True
    E. False

74. A. False
    B. False
    C. False
    D. True

75. A. True
    B. False
    C. False
    D. True
    E. True

76. A. True
    B. False
    C. False
    D. False
    E. False

77. A. True
    B. True
    C. False
    D. False
    E. False

The majority of cases are diagnosed with radiological investigations or during cystoscopy. Surgical intervention is not indicated unless there is persistent infection.

78. A. True
    B. False
    C. True
    D. True
    E. False

There is no scientific evidence that urethral caruncle predates urethral cancer.

79. A. False
    B. False
    C. True
    D. True
    E. False

An enterocoele is a herniation of the small bowel into the upper posterior vaginal wall. The levator ani muscles are important supporting structures of the pelvic organs, together with other tissues.

80. A. False
    B. True
    C. True
    D. False

Burch colposuspension is contraindicated when there is a foreshortened, scarred and immobile vagina.

81. A. False
    B. False
    C. False
    D. True
    E. False

Note the word 'irreversible'.

82. A. True
    B. False
    C. False
    D. False

GSI is the commonest form of incontinence, occurring in about 70% of female patients.

83. A. True
    B. False
    C. True
    D. False
    E. True

84. A. False
     B. False
     C. False
     D. True
     E. False

After 6 months, the treatment is associated with very little, if any, reduction in spine or hip bone density.

85. A. True
     B. False
     C. True
     D. False
     E. False

86. A. True
     B. False
     C. False
     D. False
     E. True

87. A. False
     B. False
     C. True
     D. False
     E. False

Premature ovarian failure occurs in 1–5% of women.

88. A. True
     B. True
     C. False

89. A. True
     B. True
     C. False
     D. True
     E. False

90. A. False
     B. True
     C. False
     D. True

91. A. True
    B. False
    C. False
    D. True
    E. True

92. A. True
    B. False
    C. False
    D. False
    E. False

The failure rate is between 1.4 and 4.3 pregnancies per 100 women years.

93. A. False
    B. False
    C. False
    D. True

Depot medroxyprogesterone acetate is a derivative of 17-alpha-hydroxyprogesterone. Liver enzymes have no action on DMA.

94. A. False
    B. True
    C. False
    D. True
    E. False

The secretions come from the cervix and vagina. Doderlein's bacillus is an aerobic gram-positive rod.

95. A. True
    B. True
    C. False
    D. True
    E. True

96. A. False
     B. False
     C. True
     D. False

The failure rate is about 1–3 per 1000. This figure increases when sterilization is performed at the time of Caesarean section.

97. A. True
     B. True
     C. False
     D. True
     E. False

98. A. True
     B. False
     C. False
     D. False
     E. True
     F. False
     G. False

DVT is three times greater in the left leg than in the right. It is sickle cell disease, not the trait, that has an association with venous thrombosis in pregnancy. Women with antiphospholipid antibody syndrome have a significant risk of CVA and IUGR. The average life span for platelets is 9–12 days. Heparin therapy, not warfarin therapy, may cause alopecia, thrombocytopenia and osteoporosis.

99. A. True
     B. False
     C. True
     D. True
     E. False

100. A. False
     B. False
     C. True
     D. False
     E. False

101. A. False
     B. False
     C. True
     D. True
     E. True

Diabetes mellitus influences male fertility, not diabetes insipidus. Bronchiectasis, not bronchitis, influences male fertility.

102. A. False
     B. True
     C. True
     D. False
     E. True
     F. False

If colposcopy is unsatisfactory and the smear shows severe dyskaryosis, a cone biopsy is advisable. Cervical stenosis following cone biopsy may give rise to menstrual dysfunction or dysmenorrhoea.

103. A. False
     B. True
     C. False
     D. True
     E. True
     F. False

Cerebrovascular disease is ten times more common during pregnancy and the puerperium. Approximately 60% of women with hereditary antithrombin III develop a venous thrombosis in pregnancy. There is an association between antiphospholipid antibody syndrome and phlebothrombosis. Pulmonary embolus occurs in 0.3–1.2% of all pregnancies.

104. A. True
     B. False
     C. True
     D. True
     E. False
     F. False

Granulosa cell tumours have a good prognosis and they occur at any age. They are associated with endometrial carcinoma in 0.6–6% of cases.

105. A. True
      B. False
      C. True
      D. False
      E. False
      F. True
      G. True
      H. True

Abdominal pain is present in about 90% of ectopic
pregnancies. Low levels of progesterone are more common
in ectopic pregnancies as opposed to intrauterine pregnancies.
A coexisting ectopic and intrauterine pregnancy occurs in 1 in
30 000 pregnancies.

106. A. False
      B. False

Maternal mortality is 4.5 times higher following elective
Caesarean section and 18 times higher following emergency
Caesarean section than after vaginal delivery.

107. A. False
      B. True

A recent study (Enkin) reported 58–81% vaginal delivery in a
group of women who had had two previous Caesarean
sections for non-recurrent cause.

108. A. True
      B. True
      C. False
      D. False
      E. False
      F. True
      G. False

There is a covering membrane at the apex of exomphalos.
Gastroschisis defect is almost invariably on the right of a
normal umbilical cord insertion and the male:female ratio is
similar. It is exomphalos, not gastroschisis, that is associated
with about a 50% incidence of chromosomal anomalies.

---

109. A. True
B. False
C. False
D. False
E. False

Fetal death occurs in less than 1% of cases, but there is a significant risk of cord entanglement and placental abruption.

110. A. False
B. False
C. True
D. True
E. True
F. False

Laparoscopic sterilization is not essential prior to endometrial resection, but patients should be aware of the unacceptably high risk of pregnancy after the procedure. Laparotomy may be indicated in some cases of postoperative bleeding.

111. A. False
B. True
C. True
D. True

Retroperitoneal lymph node spread is usually an early and common phenomenon.

112. A. True
B. True
C. False
D. False

Primary hypothyroidism and central precocious puberty are gonadotrophin-dependent causes of precocious puberty.

113. A. False
     B. False
     C. True
     D. True
     E. True
     F. True

Plasma progesterone of more than 30 nmol/l in the putative luteal phase is normal. Serum prolactin is unlikely to be abnormal in a patient with regular cycles.

114. A. False
     B. True
     C. False
     D. True
     E. False

Hyperprolactinaemia usually presents as secondary amenorrhoea and occurs in about 30% of those who have given birth.

115. A. False
     B. False
     C. True

Pericardial effusion is a rare presentation of the syndrome. Ovarian hyperstimulation syndrome is unlikely to occur if the corpora lutea are not stimulated.

116. A. False
     B. False
     C. True
     D. False
     E. True
     F. True

60% of the ampullary and fimbrial cells are ciliated. The fertilized egg spends 4–5 days in the tube. After one episode of PID, subsequent tubal occlusion occurs in about 12% of cases but after three attacks this rises to 75%. Ascending PID infection predominantly affects the mucosa.

117. A. False
     B. False
     C. False
     D. False
     E. False
     F. False
     G. False

All of the above are known to cause incontinence.

118. A. False
     B. True
     C. False

Sperm production takes 3 to 4 months. It is oligospermia, not azoospermia, that indicates a low sperm count.

119. A. False
     B. True
     C. True
     D. False
     E. False
     F. False

Trophoblastic tumours are more common in Asia. There is an increased risk of recurrence in subsequent pregnancies.

120. A. False
     B. True
     C. True
     D. True

Ovarian involvement is encountered in about 60% of cases. The increase in incidence is largely due to an increase in the number of diagnostic laparoscopies. Danazol (a derivative of 17-alpha-ethinyl testosterone) is not commonly used for treatment due to side-effects.

121. A. False
     B. False
     C. False
     D. True
     E. False

Serum CA 125 is raised in more than 80% of patients with ovarian cancer.

122. A. False
     B. False
     C. True

There is a reduction in the peripheral vascular resistance and cardiac output is increased during pregnancy.

123. A. True
     B. True
     C. True
     D. False

Penetration depth for the skin with the CO_2 laser is about 0.05 mm.

124. A. False
     B. False
     C. False
     D. False
     E. False
     F. False

A–F are all known causes of chronic pelvic pain.

125. A. True
     B. True
     C. True
     D. True
     E. True
     F. True
     G. True
     H. True
     I. True

126. A. False
      B. True
      C. False

5–10% of endometrial lesions may be overlooked by D&C.
Uterine perforation occurs in 0.5–1.3% of cases and excessive
bleeding occurs in less than 1%.

127. A. False
      B. True
      C. True
      D. False
      E. False
      F. False
      G. True
      H. True

Mifepristone is an antiprogestogen that is given orally. Peak
plasma concentration is reached 1–2 hours after administration.
Currently it is licensed for use in medical terminations up to
7 weeks.

128. A. True
      B. True
      C. False
      D. False

The marked decline in incidence of chromosomal
abnormalities is due to TOP. Edward's syndrome is a trisomy
18 and Patau's syndrome is a trisomy 13. AFP levels are
reduced in most chromosomal diseases.

129. A. True
      B. False
      C. False
      D. False
      E. True

NTDs are by far the commonest lesions identified. Cardiac
abnormalities can be very difficult to diagnose. Calyceal
dilatation may develop at around 30 weeks, therefore it cannot
be detected early.

130. A. **False**
      B. **False**
      C. **False**
      D. **True**
      E. **False**

Local anaesthetic is not usually required for amniocentesis. Using methylene blue is not safe in cases of twins as it is associated with multiple ileal occlusions. Culture failure occurs in about 0.5%. Amniocentesis may be used to assess haemolytic diseases and fetal lung maturity in late pregnancy.

131. A. **True**
      B. **False**
      C. **False**
      D. **True**
      E. **True**
      F. **False**

Tay–Sachs' disease, beta thalassaemia and cystic fibrosis are all autosomal recessive diseases.

132. A. **False**
      B. **False**
      C. **False**
      D. **False**
      E. **False**
      F. **False**

All the above are known to cause urge syndrome.

133. A. **True**
      B. **True**
      C. **True**
      D. **True**
      E. **False**

134. A. **False**
B. **True**
C. **False**
D. **True**
E. **True**

Significant uterine enlargement is not a contraindication to vaginal hysterectomy, but it is still considered so, traditionally, by some.

135. A. **False**
B. **False**
C. **True**
D. **False**

Imperforate hymen occurs typically in 14–16-year-old girls and there is usually amenorrhoea. Secondary sexual development is usually normal.

136. A. **True**
B. **False**
C. **True**
D. **True**
E. **False**

There is no evidence that mild endometriosis affects fertility.

137. A. **True**
B. **False**
C. **False**
D. **False**
E. **False**

There is a peripheral distribution of follicles in PCO, decreased ovarian stroma and increased ovarian volume. The changes are related to the ovaries, not the uterus.

138. A. True
      B. True
      C. False
      D. True
      E. False

Epidural analgesia is associated with hypotension and there is some evidence to suggest that it affects the duration of the second stage of labour.

139. A. True
      B. True
      C. True
      D. True
      E. True

140. A. False
      B. True
      C. True
      D. True
      E. True
      F. False

The puerperium usually includes the first 6 weeks post-delivery. Beta human gonadotrophin is negative about 2 weeks after term delivery. Only 40–50% of bottle-feeding mothers have their first period by 6 weeks postpartum.

141. A. True
      B. False
      C. True
      D. True
      E. True
      F. False
      G. False

Placental abruption is diagnosed clinically. Retroplacental clots may or may not be visualized by ultrasound scan so it is not a good discriminatory test. There is no evidence that placental abruption is commoner in patients with renal transplants.

142. A. True
     B. True
     C. True
     D. True
     E. True
     F. True
     G. False

Vacuum aspiration for termination of pregnancy is associated with a maternal mortality of 1 in 100 000.

143. A. False
     B. True
     C. True
     D. True

There is a significant increase in serum thyroxine-binding globulin in pregnancy.

144. A. False
     B. True
     C. True
     D. True
     E. False
     F. True
     G. False
     H. True

Although eclampsia has no association with smoking during pregnancy, it tends to be more severe if it does occur. It is placental abruption, not placenta praevia, that is associated with smoking during pregnancy.

145. A. True
     B. True
     C. True
     D. False
     E. False
     F. False

The Manning criteria for biophysical profile states that continuous fetal breathing movements should occur for at least 30 seconds, with no more than 6 seconds between breaths. At least three gross fetal body movements are required. Up to 30 minutes' scanning is allowed to fulfil all the test requirements.

146. A. True
   B. False
   C. True
   D. False
   E. False

In uterine inversion, the cervix usually closes and this will add to the difficulties of repositioning the uterus. Uterine hypotonia is a known risk factor in uterine inversion, but there is no racial predisposition.

147. A. True
   B. False
   C. True
   D. True
   E. True

Endometrial hyperplasia may be due to endogenous as well as exogenous hormonal stimulation.

148. A. True
   B. False
   C. True
   D. False
   E. True

Mixed mesodermal tumours contain striated muscle (rhabdomyosarcoma).

149. A. True
   B. True
   C. False
   D. False

Patients with gonadoblastomas are phenotypically female. The gonads should be removed even in unilateral lesions.

150. A. True
   B. False
   C. True
   D. False

The immature teratoma is derived from all the embryological layers. Only 1–2% of cases of benign cystic teratoma are potentially malignant.

151. A. True
B. False
C. True
D. True
E. True
F. True

152. A. False
B. True
C. False
D. True
E. True
F. False

It is potassium chloride rather than potassium iodide that is used. Actinomycin has been tried, but prolonged use is a disadvantage.

153. A. True
B. False
C. True
D. True
E. True
F. True
G. False

154. A. False
B. True
C. True
D. True
E. False

Serous adenocarcinomas comprise 40% of all malignant ovarian tumours. Hobnail cells are found in clear cell adenocarcinoma.

155. A. True
B. True
C. True
D. True
E. True
F. True

156. A. True
B. True
C. True
D. True
E. False

Early menarche usually occurs in well-nourished populations.

157. A. False
B. True
C. True
D. True
E. False
F. False

The LH/FSH ratio is raised in PCO.

158. A. False
B. True
C. True
D. False

The incidence of hyperemesis gravidarum is increased following a previous unsuccessful pregnancy.

159. A. True
B. True
C. True
D. True
E. True
F. False

160. A. True
B. False
C. False
D. False
E. True

The skin loss and scarring in congenital varicella syndrome is unilateral and segmental. The syndrome includes hypoplastic or rudimentary digits and there may be poor fetal growth.

161. A. True
     B. True
     C. False
     D. True
     E. True
     F. False

Menstrual disturbance occurs in about 20% of cases.
Mycobacteria are obligate aerobes.

162. A. False
     B. True
     C. True
     D. False
     E. False

Urine enters the bladder at a rate of 0.5–5 ml per minute.
Baseline bladder pressure increases during filling from 10 cm
to no more than 15 cm of water.

163. A. True
     B. True
     C. True

164. A. False
     B. True
     C. True
     D. True
     E. False

Bartholin's gland carcinomas are rare and account for only
1–2% of all vulval cancers.

165. A. True
     B. True
     C. False
     D. True
     E. False

The 5-year survival rate for patients with clear cell
adenocarcinoma is about 78%. Abnormal vaginal smears are
present in 80% of cases.

166. A. False
      B. True
      C. False

The age group most commonly affected is women in their 40s.
Menorrhagia and secondary dysmenorrhoea are the
commonest presenting symptoms.

167. A. False
      B. True
      C. True
      D. False
      E. True
      F. True

LHRH analogue therapy is suitable in young women.

168. A. True
      B. True
      C. True
      D. True
      E. False
      F. False

PCO and acromegaly are androgen-dependent causes of
hirsutism.

169. A. False
      B. False
      C. False

Vaginal melanoma is rare and usually presents in the lower
third of the vagina. Surgical treatment is not usually successful.

170. A. True
      B. True

171. A. False
      B. True
      C. False
      D. True
      E. True

Virilism is associated with ovarian or adrenal tumours. It is the
absence of mullerian factor that is linked with virilism.

172. A. True
     B. True
     C. False
     D. True
     E. True
     F. True
     G. False

The beta chains of the fetal haemoglobin are replaced by
gamma chains. Apparently pregnancy has no effect on
Hodgkin's disease.

173. A. True
     B. False
     C. False
     D. False

Thrombocytopenia in pregnant women can affect the fetus
in 20% of cases if the fetus becomes thrombocytopenic.
Splenectomy should be avoided in later pregnancy. The aim
should be vaginal delivery, unless there are indications for
Caesarean section in these patients.

174. A. True
     B. False
     C. True

Fragile X syndrome is the second commonest cause of mental
retardation after Down's syndrome. It affects males. With
amniocentesis, there are occasional false negative results.

175. A. False
     B. True
     C. False
     D. True
     E. True
     F. False

The deficiency in Von Willebrand's disease is in the activity of
factor VIII and the disease is an autosomal dominant condition.
The combined oral contraceptive pill may be used in this
condition.

176. A. False
B. True
C. True
D. False
E. True
F. False
G. False

Arterial disease is the main cause of death. Bone loss accelerates in the 6 to 10 years following the menopause. Socio-economic factors, race, weight and height are related to the onset of menarche. The levels of oestradiol and androstenedione are markedly reduced.

177. A. True
B. True
C. True
D. False
E. True
F. False
G. False

Poor memory, irritability and anorgasmia are related to psychological symptoms of the menopause.

178. A. True
B. False
C. True
D. True
E. True
F. True
G. True
H. True
I. True

Hyperparathyroidism is associated with secondary osteoporosis.

179. A. True
B. True
C. True
D. True
E. True
F. True

180. A. False
     B. True
     C. False
     D. True
     E. True

Vaginal dryness is a symptom of urogenital atrophy.
Dyspareunia, not dysmenorrhoea, is also a symptom.

181. A. True
     B. False
     C. True
     D. False
     E. True
     F. False
     G. True
     H. True

Tibolone has weak oestrogenic and progestogenic properties
and has a low incidence of withdrawal bleeding.

182. A. False
     B. False
     C. True
     D. True

Spermicides are usually used in conjunction with a barrier
method. Nonoxynol-9 is the most commonly used spermicide.

183. A. True
     B. True
     C. False
     D. True
     E. False
     F. True

It is important to remember that ectopic pregnancy can result
in ovarian hyperstimulation syndrome.

184. **A.** True
 B. False
 C. False
 D. False

When hyperprolactinaemia is suspected, hypothyroidism should be excluded. Dopamine agonists, not antagonists, may be used to treat hyperprolactinaemia.

185. **A.** True
 B. True
 C. False
 D. True
 E. True
 F. False

Hyperprolactinaemia, not hypoprolactinaemia, may cause secondary amenorrhoea. Hypogonadotrophic hypogonadism may cause secondary amenorrhoea, not hypergonadotrophic hypogonadism.

186. **A.** True
 B. True
 C. True
 D. True
 E. True

187. **A.** False
 B. True
 C. True
 D. False
 E. False
 F. True

Phaeochromocytoma arises from the adrenal medulla. Surgical removal of the tumour in early pregnancy results in spontaneous abortion. Increased abdominal pressure may cause a large release of catecholamines and it is ideal to perform a combined procedure of Caesarean section and removal of tumour through an elongated incision when the fetus is viable.

188. **A. True**
     B. True
     C. False

The incidence of endocervical adenocarcinoma is increasing in young women.

189. **A. True**
     B. False
     C. True
     D. True
     E. True
     F. True
     G. False

The differential diagnosis is hyperparathyroidism, not hypoparathyroidism. It is small bowel obstruction that is a differential diagnosis, not large bowel obstruction.

190. **A. True**
     B. False
     C. False

Endoscopic bladder neck suspension is indicated particularly for elderly patients. It is usually indicated for patients who have had multiple unsuccessful operations.

191. **A. False**
     B. True
     C. True
     D. False
     E. False
     F. False

Chondrodysplasia punctata is associated with warfarin usage. Warfarin does cross the placenta. Warfarin may cause microcephaly due to intracranial haemorrhages. Heparin is linked to bone demineralization in the mother, as it does not cross the placenta.

192. A. False
     B. True
     C. True
     D. True
     E. False
     F. False
     G. False

Cyanosis is not present with pulmonary stenosis. In Eisenmenger's complex, there is always an interventricular septal defect seen and cyanosis is a late feature. In patients with heart disease, both spinal and epidural anaesthetics are preferable for Caesarean section.

193. A. True
     B. True
     C. True
     D. True

Anaphylactic haemolytic anaemia occurs very rarely following absorption of the distension fluid.

194. A. False
     B. False
     C. False
     D. False
     E. False

The incidence of ovarian and endometrial cancer is reduced by 40% in women taking combined oral contraceptives. The incidence of benign breast disease, not potentially malignant disease, is reduced by 50%. The incidence of uterine fibroids is reduced by about 17% and the incidence of pelvic inflammatory disease is reduced by about 50%.

195. A. False
     B. True
     C. False
     D. True

Methyldopa is associated with a decreased head circumference. Atenolol is considered safe in pregnancy.

196. A. True
      B. True
      C. False
      D. True
      E. False

There is an increase in sex-hormone-binding globulin in patients taking the combined oral contraceptive pill. Most clotting factors are increased.

197. A. True
      B. False
      C. True
      D. False
      E. False

Exenteration is contraindicated if there is evidence of spread of the tumour outside the pelvis. Should small bowel obstruction occur following the procedure, it should be treated conservatively as there is a high mortality rate on a second laparotomy. The success rate is between 20 and 50%.

198. A. False
      B. True
      C. True
      D. True

Danazol is an isoxazol derivative of 17-alpha-ethinyl testosterone. It directly inhibits ovarian and adrenal steroidogenesis.

199. A. False
      B. True
      C. True
      D. False
      E. False

The mature cystic teratoma is a germ cell tumour. The presence of well-formed teeth occurs in a third of mature cystic teratomas. Teratoma of the testis frequently behaves in a malignant manner.

200. A. True
     B. True
     C. True
     D. True

201. A. False
     B. True
     C. False

Amenorrhoea, abdominal pain and interference with micturition are the predominant features of haematocolpos.

202. A. False
     B. True
     C. False

The chromosomal pattern in Klinefelter's syndrome is 47XXY. Gynaecomastia is a common presenting sign.

203. A. True
     B. True
     C. True
     D. True

204. A. True
     B. True
     C. False
     D. False

In Laurence–Moon–Biedl syndrome, mental retardation will be evident in infancy. Syndactyly is a recognized feature.

205. A. True
     B. False
     C. True
     D. True

Breast atrophy, not hypertrophy, is a feature of virilism.

206. A. True
    B. True
    C. False
    D. True
    E. True

Simple diffusion is a known function of the placenta.

207. A. False
    B. True
    C. True
    D. False

Relaxin inhibits rather than stimulates myometrial activity during pregnancy. Relaxin enhances sperm mobility.

208. A. True
    B. True
    C. False
    D. True
    E. True
    F. True

209. A. True
    B. False
    C. False

Alpha-chain synthesis is suppressed in alpha thalassaemia. The homozygous form is incompatible with life.

210. A. False
    B. False
    C. False
    D. False

Treatment of advanced Hodgkin's disease in pregnancy is therapeutic abortion followed by chemotherapy.

211. A. True
      B. False
      C. False
      D. False
      E. True
      F. True
      G. False

Ritodrine hydrochloride is contraindicated in all cases of
intrauterine infection. It may cause hypokalaemia, not
hyperkalaemia. It is definitely contraindicated in patients with
cardiac disease.

212. A. False
      B. True
      C. True
      D. True

The incidence of urinary calculus is less than 1% of all
pregnancies.

213. A. False
      B. True
      C. True
      D. False

Diazepam crosses the placenta and suppresses the beat-to-beat
variability. The use of magnesium sulphate may cause
hypocalcaemic tetany.

214. A. False
      B. True
      C. True
      D. True
      E. True
      F. False
      G. True

The incidence of Down's syndrome is about 1 in 700
pregnancies. Heart problems occur in 40% of cases of Down's
syndrome.

215. A. True
      B. True
      C. False
      D. True

The incidence of chorioamnionitis is higher in women delivering preterm babies.

216. A. True
      B. True
      C. True
      D. True
      E. True
      F. True

217. A. False
      B. True
      C. False
      D. True

There is a decrease in the peripheral vascular resistance and cardiac output is increased during a normal pregnancy.

218. A. False
      B. True
      C. True

Peptic ulcer is rare in the reproductive age group.

219. A. False
      B. True
      C. True
      D. True
      E. True
      F. True

Gonorrhoea in pregnancy may be asymptomatic.

220. A. True
      B. False
      C. True
      D. True
      E. True

221. A. False
 B. True
 C. False
 D. True
 E. True
 F. True
 G. True

Dichlorophen should not be used in pregnancy as it can cause severe diarrhoea.

222. A. True
 B. False
 C. True
 D. True
 E. True

Threatened abortion, not missed abortion, affects the interpretation of serum marker results.

223. A. False
 B. False
 C. True
 D. True

The incidence of craniospinal anomalies is 2–4 per 1000 births and the incidence of cardiovascular anomalies is 8 per 1000 births.

224. A. True
 B. True
 C. True
 D. False

225. A. True
 B. True
 C. False

The risk of death from obstetric haemorrhage is about 1 in 100 000 deliveries. Ligation of the internal iliac artery prevents hysterectomy in only 50% of obstetric haemorrhages and the technique needs a high degree of surgical skill.

226. A. False
      B. False
      C. False
      D. False

Partial or complete duplication of the ureter results from early splitting of the ureteric bud. The kidneys do not completely separate as a result of the intermingling of the collecting tubules. An ectopic ureter is one that opens anywhere but the trigone and ectopic ureters opening below the urethral sphincter mechanism usually become clinically and anatomically evident, producing continuous urinary incontinence.

227. A. True
      B. True
      C. False

228. A. True
      B. False
      C. True
      D. True

229. A. True
      B. False
      C. True
      D. True

Prolonged labour *per se* does not predispose to puerperal sepsis, but when there are repeated vaginal examinations, this might be a predisposing factor.

230. A. False
      B. True
      C. True
      D. False

The overall survival in stage 1 disease is over 80%. Early recurrence of cervical cancer is associated with high mortality.

231. A. True
     B. True
     C. False
     D. True

The incidence of testicular feminization syndrome is 1 in 50 000.

232. A. True
     B. False
     C. True
     D. False
     E. True
     F. False

Sarcomatous change occurs in about 0.2%. The capsule surrounding an intramural fibroid is a false one. Fibroids are composed of smooth muscle cells.

233. A. False
     B. False
     C. False
     D. False
     E. False

A–E are all recognized causes of hirsutism.

234. A. False
     B. False
     C. False

A–C all may cause hyperprolactinaemia.

235. A. True
     B. True
     C. True
     D. True

236. A. False
     B. False
     C. True
     D. True

Sarcoma botryoides is a highly malignant tumour. It is commonly seen in patients younger than 2 years old, but it may be seen at any age.

237. A. True
     B. True
     C. True
     D. True

238. A. True
     B. True
     C. True
     D. True

239. A. False
     B. False
     C. False
     D. False
     E. False
     F. False

A–F may all lead to hydrops fetalis.

240. A. False
     B. True
     C. False
     D. True

There is a great variation of nuclear sizes in the Arias–Stella reaction and the quantity of cytoplasm is usually increased.

241. A. True
     B. False
     C. False
     D. False
     E. False

Abdominal ectopic pregnancy is commoner in older women and occurs more commonly in low parity. Endometriosis is rarely reported. It may not be possible to remove the placenta and in this case methotrexate or dactinomycin in full antitumour dosage is given.

242. A. True
     B. True
     C. True
     D. True

243. A. True
     B. True
     C. True

244. A. True
     B. False
     C. True
     D. True

Patent ductus arteriosus is the commonest lesion in congenital
rubella infection. It is microcephalus, not hydrocephalus, that is
a feature.

245. A. False
     B. True
     C. False
     D. True
     E. True
     F. True

Hypocalcaemia and hyponatraemia are causes of neonatal
seizures.

246. A. True
     B. True
     C. True

The more definitive separation of the placenta following a
full-term delivery is the likely explanation for the rapid
clearance of human chorionic gonadotrophin from the
maternal bloodstream. This does not occur with miscarriages.

247. A. True
     B. True
     C. False
     D. True

The normal vaginal flora includes anaerobic, not aerobic,
streptococci.

248. A. False
     B. True
     C. False
     D. True
     E. True

Erythromycin acts mainly against gram-positive organisms and its activity is enhanced at alkaline pH.

249. A. True
     B. False
     C. False
     D. True
     E. False

Herpes gestationis develops after the fifth month of pregnancy. Spontaneous cure is expected in 100%.

250. A. True
     B. True
     C. True

251. A. False
     B. False
     C. True

In the gynaecoid pelvis, the interspinous diameter is usually widened. The pelvic arch is usually straight in the android pelvis.

252. A. True
     B. False
     C. False
     D. False

Phaeochromocytoma is rare in pregnancy. About 90% of tumours are benign in adults and alpha adrenergic blocking agents are the treatment of choice.

253. A. False
     B. False

The chances of the infant contracting infections are theoretically reduced and rooming-in is usually cheap.

254. A. False
     B. True
     C. False

The incidence of occult prolapse is unknown. Prolapsed umbilical cord is common with a long cord of greater than 75 cm.

255. A. False
     B. True
     C. True
     D. False
     E. False

In acute fatty liver of pregnancy, haematemesis is a typical feature. Maternal mortality is about 80%.

256. A. True
     B. False
     C. True
     D. False
     E. False

The most critical time for myasthenia gravis is postpartum. Scopolamine is not a safe drug to use as it masks anticholinergic drugs overdose. Transient neonatal myasthenia gravis is seen in 20–30%.

257. A. False
     B. True
     C. False
     D. False

Ovarian rupture is likely in more than 90% of cases of ovarian pregnancy. Hysterectomy is very rarely indicated.

258. A. False
     B. False
     C. False
     D. True
     E. False
     F. False
     G. False

A, B, C, E, F and G may be detected antenatally.

259. A. True
B. False
C. False
D. True
E. True

Fetal tachycardia may be due to maternal hyperthyroidism, not hypothyroidism. Fetal hypovolaemia, not hypervolaemia, may cause fetal tachycardia.

260. A. True
B. True
C. True
D. False
E. False
F. False
G. False

Cervico-oculo-acoustic syndrome is an X-linked dominant condition. Marfan's syndrome, Huntington's chorea and night blindness are all autosomal dominant conditions.

261. A. False
B. True
C. True

Levels of serum LH fall in anorexia nervosa as a result of hypothalamic suppression.

262. A. True
B. False
C. False
D. False

The soft chancre is caused by *H. ducreyi*, which is a gram-negative rod. It is characterized by a painful genital ulcer and the incubation period is short. The lesion appears in 3–5 days.

263. A. True
     B. False
     C. False
     D. True

Sarcoma of the cervix is common in postmenopausal women and there is no known association with sexual behaviour, in contrast to carcinoma of the cervix.